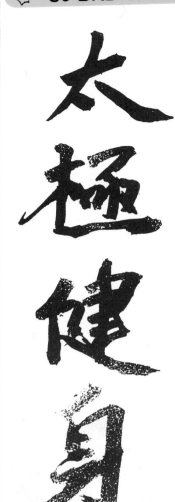

Disclaimer

The reader or readers should consult his or her physician for advice on whether or not the reader or readers should embark on the physical activity described herein. The publisher is NOT RESPONSIBLE in any manner whatsoever for any injury which may occur by following the instructions herein.

Library of Congress Catalog Card Number 89-52077

Includes index

1. Fitness exercises. 2. Sport Training. 3. Tai-ji Quan

Paperback ISBN 0-9625392-0-1

Printed in the United States of America

First paperback edition

TAI-JI FITNESS

Its Principles and Basic Training

The Way to Total Fitness

Xiaonan Zhang, Ph. D.

To my mother and father.

With grateful acknowledgment to my Tai—ji Quan teachers, friends and students from whom I learned so much. To my wife, whose love and support made this book possible.

Special thanks to my Tai—ji Quan teacher, Dr. David J. Wu, whose teaching made this work possible.

Special thanks to Dr. K. Loeffler, Dr. G. R. Burke, Ms. M. Hamermesh, Mr. J. E. Kowalski for their support in the preparation of the book.

PREFACE

In today's east Asia – China, Japan, and Singapore there are millions of people who practice Tai–ji Quan (T'ai Chi Ch'uan) as a health and fitness exercise. Many people consider Tai–ji Quan to be a useful aid in combating the debilitating effects of arthritis, heart disease and hypertension. By distilling the essence of the fitness aspect of Tai–ji Quan and eliminating the sole martial arts–related exercise, Tai–ji principles are introduced here in a more general form. My goal is to introduce Tai–ji principles and fitness training to English readers. Therefore, brief, clear and scientific writing has been chosen as the style of this book.

Ever since I began practicing Tai–ji Quan, I have seen the changes in my body, especially in the way I move. I have been considering the following questions:

1) What are the essentials of Tai–ji Quan?
2) How can I develop a set of exercises which are based on Tai–ji principles?
3) How can I reduce the learning time?
4) How can I bring Tai–ji principles to a more general and simplified form so that people can benefit from it without actually practicing Tai–ji Quan?

After many years of practice, the above ideas matured to an over–all picture. The idea of sharing my experience and introducing this wonderful and mysterious ancient Chinese wisdom to people who want to be physically and mentally fit gave me the courage to write this book. I originally wanted to write it in Chinese and then translate it into English. Because of the difference between the two cultures, I have found that it is extremely difficult to read a translated book. Even though English is not my native language, I have decided to write this book in English with the sole purpose of reaching a larger group of Western readers.

For people who are interested in the pursuit of total fitness, this book introduces Tai–ji fitness philosophy, its principles and basic training exercises. Applying the principles to your exercise will make it more enjoyable. The training is concentrated on the fundamental basis of physical fitness. As long as you move your body, you will benefit from the exercises. By following the book and through hard and persevering practice, you will find that:

1. Your general health will improve considerably.
2. Your general athletic skills will improve significantly.
3. You will achieve a fitness level beyond what any
   other fitness programs presently available can offer.
   The benefits will affect every aspect of your life.

For people who practice Tai–ji Quan or Wu–shu(Chinese martial arts), this book introduces the basic requirements to master the art. You may find that most people do not meet the requirements. The exercises are designed to overcome the most common difficulties that people encounter in learning Tai–ji Quan. Once you master the skills introduced here, you will gain a firm base, from which you may advance in the art. Many misconceptions are also clarified in this book.

If you want to be a competitive athlete, this book also introduces Tai–ji spirit and principles for you to follow. By putting some effort into the basic fundamental fitness training introduced in this book, and applying the principles to your sport, you will be able to improve your skills to a further extent.

I hope this book will help to introduce you, the reader, to the wonderful ancient Chinese sport, fitness exercises and philosophy – Tai–ji Quan.

TABLE OF CONTENTS

TABLE OF CONTENTS [continued]

TABLE OF CONTENTS [continued]

Index

LIST OF FIGURES

1. INTRODUCTION

Wu-shu (Chinese martial arts) has been developed in China over thousands of years. It is a sport which has one of the longest developing histories in the world. It was once a real competitive sport since its results meant life or death. The training methods have undergone real tests year after year. The result can not be overlooked by today's people who want to be in excellent fitness or competitive condition. The study of its principles, training and developing history will give great benefits to modern sports training and fitness exercise.

About three hundred years ago, one school of martial arts arose and gradually formed its unique distinction from other styles of martial arts. This new style is called Tai-ji Quan. It followed the principles "subduing the vigorous by the soft", "adapting oneself to the style of others" and "overcoming a force of 1000 pounds with a force of four ounces". Tai-ji represents the balance of Yin and Yang. Quan means "fist". All together, Tai-ji Quan means a boxing style that emphasizes the balance of Yin and Yang. One of the most important characteristics is that its training (the forms) consists of a set of circular, relaxed and smooth movements. The superior fighting skills of the masters of this style over other styles formed many legendary stories. The question is how and why those masters of Tai-ji Quan achieved their unmatchable skills, and what we can learn from Tai-ji principles and training methods.

Before practicing Tai-ji Quan, I was active in swimming, running, gymnastics, soccer and many other sports. I considered myself to be in good shape and in excellent physical condition. After practicing Tai-ji Quan, I realized that it requires a very high degree of fitness. I was shocked to learn that my fitness did not meet the basic requirements of Tai-ji Quan at all. My many years pursuit of fitness was mocked by Tai-ji Quan. Therefore I was determined to learn and master Tai-ji Quan.

In order to further improve my Tai-ji Quan skills, I have been trying to find a book which talks about Tai-ji basic training. So far I have not been very successful. I, therefore, always try to find the essence of the art and then invent a simple training exercise to overcome my weakness. As a result, my Tai-ji skills have improved at a very quick pace, my fitness reached a higher level, and my health improved amazingly.

Tai-ji Quan is the epitome of ancient Chinese culture. It contains a varieties of topics such as philosophy, psychology, meditation, physical exercise and martial arts. In this book, I intend to concentrate on the fitness aspect of Tai-ji Quan. You will learn some of the ways that enhance your total fitness. This will make a difference in your life. The exercises and techniques presented in this book come from my personal experiences with many setbacks and many detours. I am delighted to be able to share my own discovery of Tai-ji fitness principles with you, and introduce some of the basic training, Tai-ji exercises, that I developed. The purpose of introducing Tai-ji training is not to replace your current fitness training but to enrich and enhance your fitness training program.

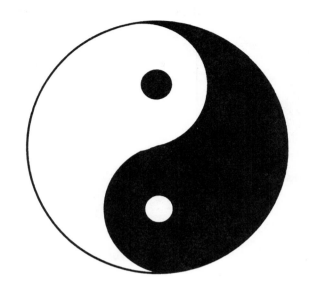

2. BASIC PRINCIPLES

In this section, I will introduce basic Tai–ji fitness principles. Since I benefited from my Tai–ji Quan practice, I have been trying to explain, for myself, why those things happened. Why did those changes take place? I hope my theory will act as a challenge and stimulus to you. You will evolve your own theory and will try to disprove my theory. At least, in this way, you will be interested in the issues and questions raised here.

Some discussions in this section are related to Tai–ji Quan. If you have no knowledge about Tai–ji Quan, you may skip those discussions.

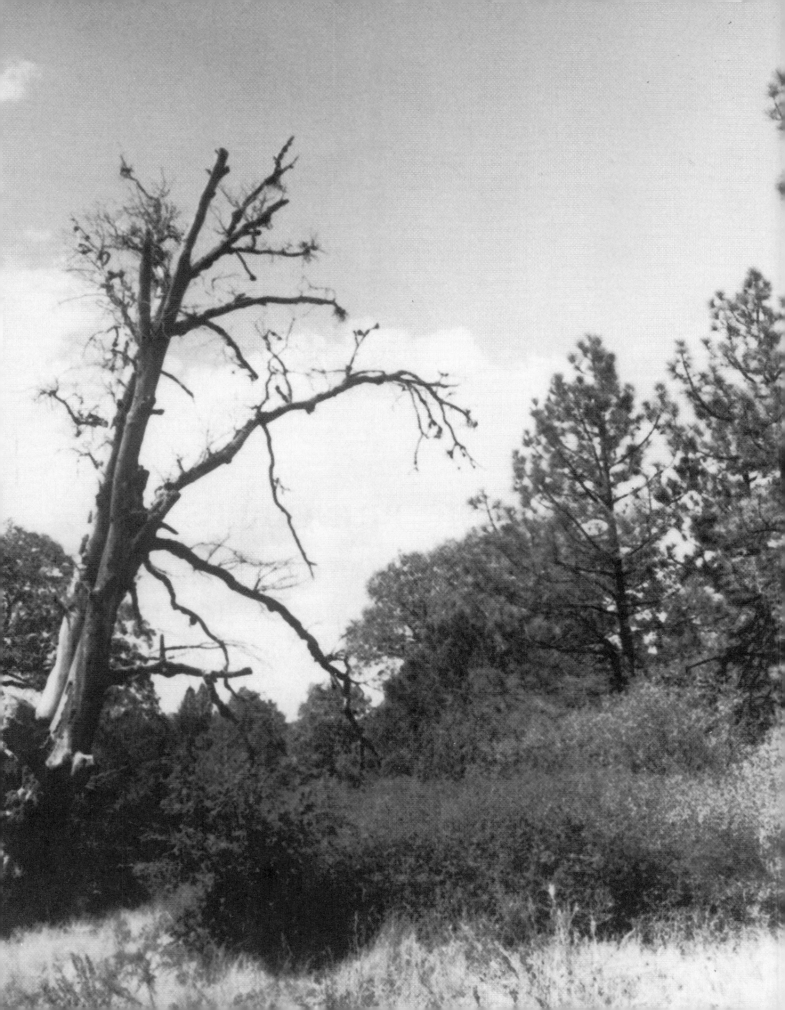

Philosophy of Tai—ji

I enjoy learning, studying and discussing the philosophical aspects of Tai—ji Quan. The Confucian, Buddhist and Taoist philosophies play very important roles in the development of Tai—ji Quan. Among them, Taoism has the most strong influence to Tai—ji Quan. Taoist philosophy is simple: Study the natural order of things and work with it rather than against it. You may have heard the words "I—Ching," "Tao Te Ching" and "Yin—Yang" and so on. They are generally subtle and abstract. Probably because of this, many people get intimidated by Tai—ji philosophy and are repelled from getting to know it. It is my intention to illustrate Tai—ji principles as scientifically as possible in this book. As an introductory book, I therefore will discuss only one aspect of Tai—ji philosophy, flexibility, in this section.

"People are born tender and flexible.
At death, they are hard and stiff
Green plants are tender and lively.
At death, they are withered and dry.

Therefore the hard and the stiff are the companions of death
The tender and the flexible are the companions of life.

Thus an army without flexibility never wins.
A tree that is unbending is easily broken.

The hard and stiff is inferior
The soft and flexible is superior. "

—Lao—tze

Lao-tze the author of "Tao Te Ching" said that more than two thousand years ago. The importance of physical flexibility is understood by many people today. For example, we know that a person who has poor spine flexibility is prone to have back injuries. What Lao-tze said here possesses a much broad meaning. In order to understand the principle, let us consider the case of a small young tree and a big old tree. To keep balance (erect) does not necessarily mean they have to be straight up rigidly, since this type of balance is stiff and inflexible. We know that when a strong wind comes, the small tree will bend, while the big tree will break. The small tree has better flexibility, or a bigger range of motion, while the big tree has poor flexibility, or small range of motion. In terms of mechanical physics, the range of motion that can be described by Hooke's law for the big tree is small. In other words, the elasticity of the big tree is not as good as the small tree. Therefore, when a strong wind comes, the small tree will bend, but the big tree will break. The larger the range of motion, the better the balance. But there is one very important thing that needs to be pointed out: elasticity. If a tree has a very big range of motion, when it is pushed to one side, it stays there rather than going back to its balanced position. This is not the range of motion we want. More precisely speaking, what we really want is the range of elastic motion. The elasticity here means the ability to recover back to a balanced position.

Applying Lao-tze's principle to people's general health, it should be interpreted as the following:

A healthy person is a person who has balance and flexibility in all aspects.

For example, a person under normal circumstances may seem fine. He may not have seen a doctor for some time. He may consider himself in good healthy condition. If he becomes sick due to change of schedule, or jetlag from travel, or an abrupt temperature change, he is not considered to be healthy because his flexibility is poor. He needs to improve his flexibility in this aspect. This means that he needs to improve his health such that he is able to maintain a good healthy body with a big temperature change, or staying up late a couple of nights. A truly healthy person should be able to change his body function with the environment accordingly. In other words, there is no absolute balance point, the balance point should change as the external condition changes. To put it concisely, be in harmony with nature.

Some experts define illness as "departure from the normal." This theory is only partially correct. If the departure is temperate, dynamic, and within the range of elastic motion, it would not necessarily be bad. If the departure is fixed, out of the range of elastic motion, then, of course, this is no good. So it is a flexibility problem or a range of elastic motion problem.

Relaxation

Many people are interested in Tai-ji Quan because of its wonderful relaxation and tension relief effect. Without tension, life will be a lot more enjoyable. Once your tension is released, your internal energy will flow unimpeded throughout your body. Your health is therefore improved.

Notice your reaction toward a challenge. Muscles all over your body become tense, opposite sets of muscles push against each other. Instead of facing the challenger with an alert mind and well prepared body, you have started fighting with yourself.

Recall what happened when you were angry, your stomach twisted, and you felt very bad inside. Here again you harmed yourself but could not help doing so. Tai-ji training will enable you to end these internal conflicts. It will improve your life physically and psychologically. Physical and mental well-being can thus be obtained.

What is the difference between Tai-ji relaxation and other forms of relaxation? Tai-ji relaxation is different from the relaxation of meditation or similar forms. Tai-ji relaxation is achieved through movements. It is dynamic. It is sports or martial arts oriented. Its essence is efficiency. One is required to relax all unnecessary muscles as the body moves.

Isolating any part of the body from other parts is a very important part of Tai-ji training. It is a basic skill to achieve higher efficiency. We will examine some of the effects of the isolation skill in fitness and sports.

Generally, most people tend to tense the muscle in larger sets and in pairs. For instance, when asked to tense the shoulder, the elbow is tensed as well. One can not tense the shoulder and keep the elbow relaxed. Or when one shoulder becomes tense due to a need to use force, the other shoulder becomes tense also. In the case of two bones which are connected by a joint (Fig. 2–1), when a force is exerted to one section, if the joint is stiff, the other section of the bone will move as well. But if the joint is very relaxed, the other section will not be affected. The relaxation of the joint isolates the upper section from the lower section. This is the isolation effect.

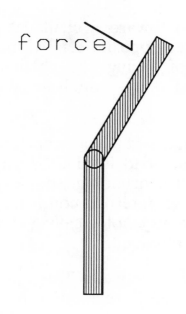

Figure 2–1 Isolation Concept

Tai–ji Quan emphasizes isolated relaxation based on its martial art applications. According to Newton's first law, force is equal to mass times acceleration. The bigger the mass is, the bigger the force becomes. The bigger the acceleration is, the bigger the force becomes. The mass of a person in a martial art application changes dramatically. This adds additional complication to the biomechanical study of sports. The ability to relax or tense any joint individually gives one control of the mass involved in a process. For example, when a person has his arm raised to shoulder level, if another person pushes his forearm, he can react in many ways:

1. Relax the elbow so that the other person only deals with the mass of the forearm.
2. Relax the shoulder and tense elbow so that the other person only moves the arm (deals with the mass of arm).
3. Relax the waist and tense arm and elbow so that the other person only makes the waist rotate an angle (deals with upper body mass).
4. Relax legs so that the coming kinetic energy is stored as potential energy in the leg muscles (deals with upper body and some leg mass).
5. Tense the related joints and direct the coming force to ground so that the other person is pushing the ground (mass equals infinity).

Tai-ji Quan practitioners make this truly an art. When you practice push-hand (a kind of sparring exercise) with a master, sometimes he is light, sometimes he is heavy, and sometimes he becomes as rigid as a stone wall. This all comes from the manipulation of relaxation and tension in joints, muscles and body position. The mass involved changes constantly. This tells us that weight lifting can not provides all that martial arts require, since the weight lifting deals with constant mass or weight.

Tai-ji exercises also teach you how to isolate your internal organs so that the internal relaxation can be achieved. The abdomen moving and the rib expanding exercises are two examples. Cultivating your body through practice of Tai-ji exercises, you will have a relaxed and alert unity of mind and body. You will be always ready to confront a challenge, or a great danger.

To what extent does "relaxed" mean in Tai-ji Quan? The Tai-ji classic treatises have described as: "When a feather is added to your arms, it should be felt for its weight." Being able to relax also leads us to high sensitivity. It is a common experience among Tai-ji practitioners that during the performance of Tai-ji Quan, the resistance of air can be sensed as we sense the water resistance in swimming. It is difficult to give an academic explanation. I hope the following story will answer the question more or less:

A master was able to keep a sparrow which was standing on his arm from flying away. He was able to accomplish this because his arm was relaxed such that every time the bird tried to push off his arm to gain initial speed for take–off, his arm dropped. The bird could not gain the initial speed for take–off. Thus the bird was prevented from flying away.

Efficiency

Tai–ji Quan emphasizes efficiency. The Tai–ji classic treatises have described as "deflecting a thousand pounds force with a trigger force of four ounces." If we want to actually do it, applying the lever principle, we need a long arm that has to be 3000 times longer than the short arm. This is impossible. Therefore, the slogan only indicates the attitude that Tai–ji practitioners should have toward efficiency. It does not mean that we do not need to develop our strength to be a good Tai–ji martial artist. When practicing Tai–ji Quan, you are asked to relax each part of your body separately, so that you know which muscles are needed to carry out the movement, and relax all the others. This is apparently already very difficult. Yet it is still not good enough. You must also use the muscles needed with minimum effort to do the work. Tai–ji exercises introduced in this book will teach you how to be a person of efficiency and productivity.

In order to understand this principle, I found a simple exercise which demonstrates the principle clearly. For the effectiveness of this exercise, you are encouraged to carry out the following exercise before continuing reading.

Stand still with feet shoulder width apart, then squat down as quickly as possible. After you have tried this, you may have the following experiences:

1. You may feel a crack in your knee or hip joints. This is due to incorrect posture.

2. Please do this a couple of times and feel all the muscle groups involved in the process. You may then discover that you contract your hamstrings in order to squat.

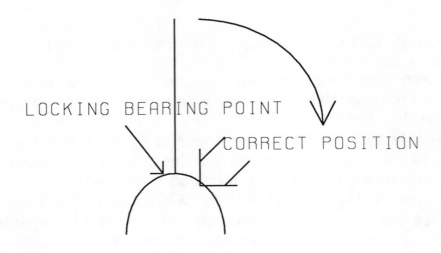

Figure 2-2 Illustration for Correct Joint Position

The first thing you can do to improve your speed is to correct your posture. The reason you hear a crack in your joints is that you position your bearing point in the locked side of the joints (Fig. 2-2). To squat, the joint has to go up hill a little bit, then slide downward. The correct posture is to bend your knees slightly and keep the spine and tail bone straight so that the bearing points are in the bending side of the joints. The latter is more difficult to do, but this does not mean that the body has to be stiff as to have no agility. You may then try to repeat the exercise. After a couple of tries, you will find that the crack or jerk in the joints has disappeared. Now you have learned one of the posture principles required in Tai-ji Quan. While practicing Tai-ji, this principle should be maintained.

Next, you should try to minimize the contraction of the hamstrings, so that by relaxing the muscle, you are able to squat down effortlessly, allowing gravity to do the work. You should observe that it is actually faster than the old way, because if you use extra strength to support your body, you have to first overcome that strength by using the opposite muscle. The tenser your muscles are, the slower they react. The most importance point is that it is not efficient.

An American young man practiced many different martial arts for many years, and had toured east Asia with unbroken records. He visited Beijing, and met a Tai-ji Quan Master Feng Zhi-qiang in the early 80s. Master Feng was over 60 year old at that time. The young man first practiced a few forms he learned and then asked Master Feng for advice. Master Feng gave a simple comment "float." The young man then had a contest with the master. With only one approach, he was lifted and thrown to over 10 feet away.

What did Master Feng mean by "float" ? The opposite word is "sink". If one learns Tai-ji Quan from a good teacher, he will be told "sink" many times. In this country, many teachers do not even mention it. A good teacher mentions "sink" because he was taught the same by his teacher. He knew what "sink" should look like because he saw how his master practiced. What is "sink"?

Let us analyze the squat exercise, you should find that when you are able to use the minimum strength to support your body, and relax all other muscles, you gain the fastest speed and the least effort to squat. While you stand with the knees slightly bent, your body actually fluctuates between the boundary of rise and sink. The feeling of "sink" comes. This is the "sink." Once you master the "sink" skill, you should notice that you can raise your body quickly as well. That is an important skill you need to master in order to follow through Tai-ji practice properly.

I am sure that the young man's skills were very good. The weakness Master Feng pointed out was a very fundamental requirement in Tai-ji Quan. So what stops him from being further advanced is nothing fancy but a very basic skill. That is one of the characteristic of Tai-ji training — working on the fundamentals.

In virtually every Wu-shu style, static stance training is adopted as a basic training to improve lower body strength. There is another benefit. By standing still for an hour or more, you eventually get so tired that you are forced to learn to use minimum strength. In this way, efficient stance is learned. One thing that differentiates Tai-ji from other styles is that Tai-ji emphasizes "sink" in movement rather than merely in static stance. Tai-ji efficiency is dynamic.

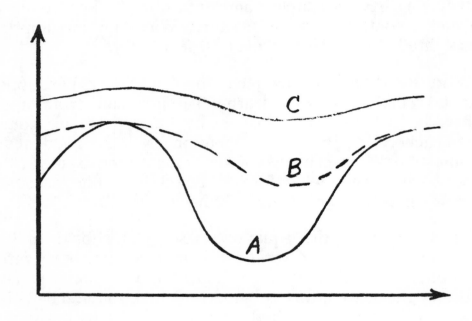

Figure 2-3 Dynamic Efficiency Concept

Fig. 2-3 illustrates the Tai-ji efficiency concept graphically. The vertical axis is the intensity of a muscle in executing a specific movement. The horizontal axis is time. The line A presents the tension needed to execute the movement of a muscle. For many people, muscle tension changes as the curve C. They think they can get things done quickly and efficiently by tensing the muscles. A skilled person may execute the movement as in the curve B. A

Tai-ji person executes the movement as in the curve A.

There are commonly two obstacles that prevent people from doing things efficiently as in the curve A. First, they can not relax muscles to that degree (bottom of the curve). Secondly, they can not relax and tense in a short period of time. Tai-ji and other exercises such as Yoga will all be able to help you to overcome the first obstacle. Only Tai-ji exercises provide the training to shorten the muscle relaxation and the muscle contraction time and improve dynamic efficiency. When you practice Tai-ji exercises, you have to be relaxed, on the other hand, you also have to carry out the physical movements. Each part of your body constantly changes from the relaxed state to the tense state. Eventually, the muscle contraction and the muscle relaxation time becomes very short. Two exercises that focus on this aspects will be discussed in the section 3, "Use of Gravity".

Many Tai-ji masters use the phrase, "Do not use force," in their teaching. What do they really mean? If they do not use force, how can they knock down their opponents? It does not make sense. Actually, what they mean is to use the minimum energy, or not to use extra force. Precisely speaking, the phrase should be "Be dynamically efficient."

Flexibility

Flexibility is one of the factors which influence agility. It represents the ability of joints to move smoothly through their maximum range of motion. How do you increase your flexibility? Flexibility is increased by stretching. Stretching may be done either ballistically or statically. Ballistic stretching involves a bouncy type of stretch, such as touching the floor with your hands in a jerky fashion. Static stretching involves a holding a stretched position for a certain period. Static stretching is recommended by exercise experts. Because it does not activate the stretch reflex. It involves less danger of exceeding the limits of your muscle.

What is the stretch reflex? When you stretch a muscle, it automatically contracts. The intensity of the contraction depends upon the suddenness and intensity of the stretch. The more intense the stretch is, the greater the stretch reflex becomes. Stretch reflex is very important in sports. For example, in tennis, during the overhead serve, the backward stretching of the extensor muscle causes a quick and powerful contraction which allows the arm to quickly begin its thrust forward.

Tai-ji stretching is somewhere between the ballistic stretching and the static stretching. Tai-ji stretching is done naturally in slow, even, circular and smooth Tai-ji movements. In the beginning, you can practice with a moderate circle size. As you gain mastery, you may then increase the size of the circles. As you gradually increase the size of the circles, stretching is executed at the same time. Tai-ji stretching is dynamic stretching. Dynamic stretching is more practical since it is this type of flexibility that people use in sports and daily activities. Because Tai-ji stretching is performed in a slow fashion, it is safer to practice.

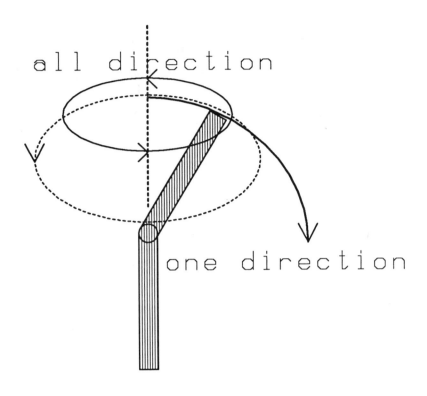

all direction

one direction

Figure 2-4 Diagram of Stretching Concept

Fig. 2-4 shows the Tai-ji stretching concept. The common stretching is done in a single direction, and working straight forward to the full range of motion (shown in bold line). Tai-ji stretching is done by working around the full range of the directions circle, then gradually increasing the angle toward the full range of motion. Please refer to the "leg stretching" exercise for details.

When moving in a circular fashion, for each set of muscles involved, there is always a half circle stretching it and the other half circle using its stretch reflex. Please notice that the natural stretch reflex may go in a different pattern, the smooth circle requires a control over the stretch reflex. Tai-ji training promotes controlled stretch reflex. Instead of looking

19

at the final result, Tai-ji people always work on the process of each action. Because they consider that success is merely a corollary of a correct process. The stretch reflex can be utilized for many movements in sports. Each sport has a particular need. Learning to modify a natural process – the stretch reflex for your own particular use is one of the important skills in Tai-ji. Two examples are introduced in the Tango walk and the waist twisting exercises, respectively. We should develop this as a life-long habit.

In sports, most injuries such as sprains do not come from one direction, it often comes from the direction where the muscles are weak. Therefore, Tai-ji exercises are excellent for sports injury prevention. Static stretching reduces the elasticity of muscles. Therefore, it is not for competitive sports. For example, some Karate people practice static stretching so that they can kick high, but their kicks became very weak and less effective.

Coordination

The importance of coordination, and its dependence upon flexibility have been mentioned by experts in many books. But in all the books, the flexibility exercise is solely for flexibility, the strength exercise is solely for strength, and the stretching is solely for stretching. I have not seen a general coordination exercise.

In Tai-ji Quan practice, coordinations are required through out the whole exercises. The principle is "One moves, all move". The materials in this aspect in Tai-ji Quan is very rich. For example, coordination of hands and eyes, hands and feet, legs, shoulders and hip, elbows and knees, internal and external and so on. In this book, most of the exercises are designed to train one or few particular parts of body. As a general and an important rule, you are encouraged to get every part of your body involved.

In today's fitness exercises, some people try very hard to invent an exercise to train a specific part of body. Tai-ji approach is to improve our body as a whole. The Tai-ji approach is the same as the traditional Chinese medicine approach which treats the body as a system. This is also why Tai-ji Quan has its healing and rejuvenating effects. Just think about how many movements we generally do at home or at work that use only one muscle. The answer is probably none. External coordination enhances the internal harmony of our body. The training of coordination of internal and external is the most important and unique part of Tai-ji Quan. You will be exposed to it in section 4.

The circular movements require very good coordination, because circular movements generally require more muscle groups working together than others. Many degenerated muscles in our body are vitalized. The smoothness requires a very good cooperation between various sets of muscles. Therefore, Tai-ji exercise provides an excellent training for coordination.

Concentration

Concentration is another important factor in life and sports. It ties closely with consistency. Tai–ji exercises are also an excellent way to improve your ability to concentrate. When you practice Tai–ji, always pay attention to your body, think the following examples:

1) Do I do this efficiently?
2) Do I do the circles smoothly?
3) Gee! I use this part of my body too much, I should use other parts of body also, or use my body as a whole.
4) How is my heart function? My body is not ready for severe exercises yet. I should wait for a while.

It is like playing chess. You have to know each of your chessman before you pay attention to your opponent. You are not asked to think of yourself all the time. In the beginning, you are asked to do so, in order to gain a very important skill of Tai–ji total fitness, self–awareness. Another way to puts this is to gain the unity of mind and body. After you know yourself very well, then you may pay attention to something else. Running with headphones on, or riding a stationary bicycle while watching TV or reading a newspaper, are not recommended. If you do not pay attention to yourself while doing exercises, when your body tells you "you are hurting me!", you would not know. If you do not respect your body, your body will not respect you. You will have problems.

As you practice the exercises, your ability to concentrate improves. You will actually not only improve your concentration ability in sports, but also benefit in your daily life.

Control and Adaptability

Many things we do require complicated body movements for which our body is not designed. For example, in baseball, in order to hit a ball hard and accurately, we have to coordinate our hands, wrists, arms, waist, legs ... for various heights and speeds of the coming ball. There are many examples like this. How can we increase our control ability generally? The circular movements in Tai-ji train you to be familiar with various positions and various movements of body naturally. The even speed and the smooth circle requirements in Tai-ji trains our control ability. The word "even" refers to the smoothness in change of speed. The word "smooth" refers to the roundness of the circles. Do not overlook the simple exercises introduced in this book. To follow the principles requires tremendous control. Having good self-control not only benefits our health, our fitness, and our sports, but also benefits our life. By practcing Tai-ji, you will improve the ability to contain your emotion under pressure, or even provoked.

Another factor in sports is adaptability by which I mean the ability to be in harmony with others. One of the characteristics of Tai-ji Quan is "adapting oneself to the style of others". Tai-ji Quan emphasizes adaptability. Adaptability is actually a different version of the range of motion or flexibility problem. For example, in ping-pong, your opponent may suddenly return a fast ball or slow ball. If you can not adjust quickly enough, you will return the ball too low or too high. The slowness and evenness in Tai-ji trains your ability to adjust your speed in a precise manner. After you can practice Tai-ji exercise in a slow and even fashion with ease, you will find that your adaptability increases. Some people having learned a self-defense technique, have difficulties in applying it effectively. They blame their opponents being faster, taller, or heavier and so on. The real problem is poor adaptability.

Many people I know say "I have no patience to practice Tai-ji. It is too slow." They would like to win in a short period of time, for instance, playing tennis. But when their opponent's tempo changes they often fail to response properly. My words to those friends are that if you really want to win, to improve your skills in your sport, go practicing Tai-ji.

Be a Child

Please observe how a child does a thing. For example, how he tries to reach a toy on a table. Note his concentration. Or on an another occasion, observe how he lifts a heavier box. Note how he uses his whole body to do it. And observe how he looks around in a new place. He has no intention to miss any of the things within his sight. Observe how babies breath, they use abdominal breathing. As we grow older, our breath become shallower. We adults often forget what we can do in our childhood. Tai-ji Quan and Tai-ji exercises train us to be natural, in other words, to be a child.

For many techniques introduced in this book, you may find that you do them naturally with no consciousness. If you have to against your natural body position to do it, no matter how great other people claim this exercise is, it is not a Tai-ji exercise. The way of Tai-ji is the way to be natural.

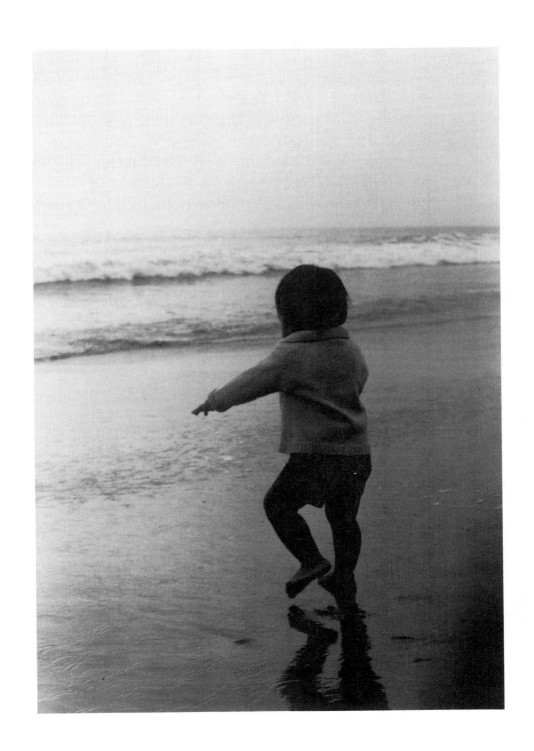

Posture

The way a person stands, walks and sits not only affects the balance in different body parts but can also cause problems in the body. The entire body works together as a system. Imbalance in one part can cause a corresponding imbalance in another. For example, a protruding pelvis may cause leg or feet problems. Standing and walking properly not only makes you look better, but also helps maintain good health.

If you read any available book about "Tai-ji Quan", you will find that there are pages of requirements you need to follow, with instructions that are difficult to understand. I think many Tai-ji followers also share the same frustration. One thing I can tell you that will make you feel better is that it is very hard for me, a Chinese, to understand the Chinese books.

If you go to a Tai-ji class, most of teachers give many strict requirements to show their knowledge and superiority. I have a completely different view point. Suppose a student comes to learn Tai-ji, and he has a stiff spine, then no matter how many times he is taught the correct posture, he will not be able to learn it, because he only has one spine position. I teach my students to increase flexibility first so that later they are able to choose from many postures. Then they discover that the most comfortable posture is the right posture. It comes naturally. Philosophy comes into the picture here. A good posture does not come from a so-called correct posture but from a good range of motion around the so-called correct posture. The bigger the range of elastic motion is, the more dynamic posture becomes, and the better your posture becomes. In fact, the correct posture varies from one situation to another. Many people I know have learned Tai-ji Quan for some time, and they still do not have the right posture. I hope this discussion gives some direction.

Mechanics of Tai—ji

In order to demonstrate the mechanics of Tai—ji, let us consider the volleyball case with which I believe most of us are familiar. To get a ball and pass it to desired position, there are three phases as shown in Fig 2—5.

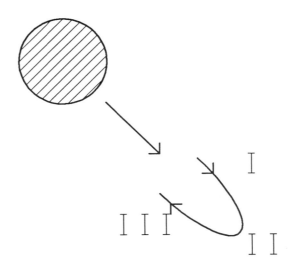

Figure 2—5 Volleyball Mechanism

Phase I — Yield phase: The person should make contact to the ball with his hands relaxed, meanwhile slow the ball down evenly. A skilled person may execute this without a sound.

Phase II — Transformation phase: Reverse the direction of the ball.

Phase III — Acceleration phase: Accelerate the ball evenly so that the ball will get to the desired place.

Now let us analyze the case. In the yield phase, if hands and arms are not relaxed but stiff at the time of contact, the ball will bounce back in a random direction. If the yield is not even, the ball will loose contact with the hands, as a result, the ball will not be passed to the desired position. The relaxation of hands actually results in longer contact time and better handling. Note here the longer time is relative to the time of stiff hands handling, certainly not a carry. Therefore, the ball must be yielded evenly with relaxed hands and arms.

In the transformation phase, the goal is to send the ball back. The moving direction of the ball must be changed. Of course, a curve is the best and the easiest way to transform the moving direction of the ball. Therefore, smooth circular movement must be used.

In the acceleration phase, to send the ball to a desired location, a relative longer contact time is needed. In terms of physics, to send the ball out requires work. The work equals time multiplied by force. For a given force, the longer time, the further distance. But if the ball is not accelerated evenly, it is suddenly accelerated in the beginning, then the ball will leave the hands right away. This, of course, is not what we want. Therefore, acceleration must be done evenly.

Now that we have gone through the volleyball analysis, the basic Tai–ji Quan movements follows the same principle described above. The only difference is that Tai–ji Quan is a martial art. The ball in the volleyball case becomes a fierce punch, kick or attack from other portion of body. The mass is heavier. Hands and arms are just not enough to handle the force. We have to use our whole body to execute the three phases. Thus in Tai–ji Quan, the three phases in the volleyball case become yield phase, neutralization phase and counter–attack phase, respectively. In order for you to understand these three phases, let us consider the case in which I react to an opponent's quick and strong push.

Phase I – Yield phase: When the push is coming toward me, to avoid losing my balance and getting injuries, I keep my body relaxed. If my body is stiff, I will be pushed off balance easily. This is one of the reasons why Tai-ji Quan is practiced in a relaxed manner. Similarly, in volleyball practice, if I use stiff fingers to hit a coming ball, I may hurt my fingers. Since my body is relaxed, after the contact, my body will move in the same direction that the on coming push moves. Instead of moving against the push, maintaining the contact and following it, this is called yield. During the yield phase, because of the contact, I will be able to sense the speed and the power of the push, then I will gradually transform to the next phase – the neutralization phase.

Phase II – Neutralization phase: Regardless of how strong the push is, if I exert a force perpendicularly to its direction, this will give me the easiest way to deviate the push. So I will use a circular motion to change my direction to the perpendicular direction, and neutralize the push. This is similar to the transformation phase in the volleyball case. After the neutralization, basically the coming force has been deviated to a different direction, so that I am out of danger. I then can go to the next phase.

Phase III – Counter-attack phase: After I neutralize the push and before my opponent relaxes his arms, I will finish my neutralization phase and turn my body to the direction facing him, my force will be exerted to his body through his arms. This is the counter-attack.

The whole process is actually done in a continuous and quick circular motion. The execution requires the skill of a smooth and small circular motion of my body. This is one of the reasons why Tai-ji Quan trains the circular movements so rigorously. The distinction of the different phases discussed here is for the purpose of illustration.

Slow and Fast

The word – "slow" has always been used to characterize Tai-ji Quan. From the above discussions, we understand the importance of slowness in Tai-ji practice. The slowness of Tai-ji exercises offer a great way to achieve high level self-control, confidence and physical strength.

How slow is adequate for beginners? Some people come to learn Tai-ji Quan from a master. The master performs at a very slow speed, they follow in the same speed. Because of their lower degree of self-control and lack of physical strength, their slow performance is accompanied by intermittent stops. This is not adequate. The proper speed for beginners should be the speed at which fluency can be maintained. By which I mean, you can practice the forms or the exercises in a continuous, fluent and non-stop manner. Once your body starts to move, every part of your body should move, there should not be a single stop in any part of your body. After many years of Tai-ji Quan, I have found that I can practice Tai-ji Quan very slowly and enjoy it. This requires a very high degree of self-control, relaxation and concentration. For beginners, emphasizing the slowness will not have the expected result. The appropriate approach toward slowness is to start in a moderate speed, gradually work on the slowness, while maintaining all other requirements.

What I just described is only one side of Tai-ji fitness. In this side, by pursuing the slowness, one will go to the meditation aspect of Tai-ji Quan. The joy of Tai-ji lies in this slowness. One gains tolerance, patience and endurance. These are all valuable assets in our lives.

There is another side of Tai-ji Quan which is not often discussed. Tai-ji Quan and Tai-ji exercises can also be practiced fast. Because of its strict requirements, most people do not get to the stage where they are qualified to practice fast. Many people think Tai-ji Quan has to be performed very slowly.   This is a misunderstanding and a very popular one.   In actuality, according to traditional Tai-ji Quan training, after you master the forms, you will be asked to practice fast.

The correct approach toward fastness is to increase speed after the basic skills have been mastered in slow motion.   By that time, your self-awareness have reached a higher level where you will be able to tell whether the requirements are still kept.   If you find any violation of the requirements, such as efficiency or smoothness, stop right away.   Go back to the speed where all the requirements can be kept and continue to practice.   Going back and forth this way until you are able to do the exercises at a high speed.   Agility is thus achieved.

Agility depends upon two key aspects.   One is physical skill.   The other is mental skill.   The key to physical agility skill lies in the mastery of fast, smooth and small circular movements in three-dimensions.   The key to mental agility skill lies in relaxation, sensitivity, self-awareness and self-control.

As speed increases, the stretch reflex becomes more and more important.   The principle described in the flexibility section should be strictly followed.   If you happen to know a person who is good in Tai-ji Quan, you may find that he has a very springy body.   The key to the springy body is proper training which involves the stretch reflex.

Straight and Curved

So far, I have mentioned the word "circular" many times. Do Taijists move in straight lines? The answer is "yes". A straight line is nothing but a curvature that has a big radius. Some people have the question "how can one defense oneself with circular movements?" The use of circular movements in Tai-ji training does not mean that Taijists use curved punch. In fact, a good straight punch is made of many circular movements of different parts of body. The word "circular" here does not mean an absolute spherical curve only. It has a broad meaning which includes a variety of different curves. Some of the details are discussed in the exercise "Figure 8 Shifting".

As you practice Tai-ji exercises, in order to know whether the curvature is smooth or not, your self-awareness is developed, in order to bring your body back to the smooth curve, the skill of fine body adjustment is learned.

The proper approach of circular movements is the follows: 1) Start with a moderate size to learn control, coordination and self-awareness; 2) Increase the size of the circles to improve flexibility and limb extensibility; 3) Decrease the size of the circles to increase your agility.

Strength

There are two types of strength exercises that are commonly discussed. One is isometric exercises. This type of exercises is static and is done with no motion. The other is isotonic exercises. This type of exercises is dynamic and is executed in motion. In this type of exercises, change of muscle's length is involved. Tai–ji strength exercises are somewhere in between. It is practiced in motion but very slow motion.

Tai–ji strength is achieved through its circular and slow movements. As we pursue the slowness of the movements, we are not only training our muscles but also our control ability, our flexibility and coordination. Unlike the muscles gained from weight lifting, strength obtained from Tai–ji training is well–controlled and flexible. In Chinese, this type of physical strength is called "jin" (skilled force). The strength which is less controlled and less flexible is called "zhuo–li" (dull force). I do not oppose the weight lifting approach. I do weight lifting myself too. The difference is in the techniques used. The circular push–up exercise is an example.

On the muscle strength aspect, we should have balanced muscles. For example, there should be a balance between hamstrings and quadricepts. On the internal and external aspect, for most people, their internal muscle strength is very weak compared to their external muscle strength. The difference is far out of proportion. Therefore, we need to develop our internal muscles. Tai–ji Quan emphasizes the internal muscle training. The basic development of internal muscle strength will be discussed in detail in section 4.

Some people have a desire to increase their strength, so they lift weights. Instead of overdeveloping the muscles and having troubles to keep the muscles firm, you may increase your strength from other perspectives which are coordination and efficiency. After practicing Tai-ji exercises and gaining some coordination and efficiency, you may find that your strength increases. For some people, after they have built their muscles, they still do not seem to be satisfied. This is because what they really looking for is stamina or energy. Being energetic is not the same as being able to lift 200 pounds. Due to their poor self-awareness, they could not realize that it is due to weak internal strength, so they keep building more external muscles. This goes in a vicious cycle. A weak internal strength has to support a much bigger external appearance. They get tired more easily. By practicing the internal training exercises, you will gain internal strength. After the internal strength is balanced with your external strength, you will become energetic and strong from inside.

Beauty of Tai-ji

When Tai-ji Quan is performed by a master, its rhythmic and coordinated movement reaches such a state of harmony that it is like a form a dance. So some people do practice Tai-ji Quan as a form of a dance. When they practice, they pay their attention to the external looks. They care about how other people think about their movements. When a real Tai-ji master practices the form, he pays all his attention to himself such that every part of his body is in harmony. The beauty is only a by-product, not the goal he pursues. That is the distinction between Tai-ji Quan and dance or calisthenics. If you practice Tai-ji Quan for performance, you will neither benefit much from Tai-ji, nor be good at it.

In today's world, many people are interested in fitness. There are many fitness centers and fitness contests. Competitors show their big muscles on stage in still postures. There is another beauty. In China, in early morning, people go to the parks to do exercises. There you may come across an old man who has brisk steps, a healthy complexion, a sonorous voice and a self-assured demeanor. The beauty comes from the practice of Tai-ji Quan or other traditional exercises. Personally, I put this type of beauty above muscle beauty.

Benefit of Tai—ji Training

The benefits of the Tai—ji training are marvelous. Tai—ji training provides us with higher efficiency, better health and better physical and mental well—being. One of the reason for better health, I think is as follows:

In order to be efficient, even, slow and circular in Tai—ji practice, we have to control each part of our body very well. How do we control? We have to control each part of our body through our nervous system. Through the pursuit of Tai—ji fitness, we are able to improve our nervous system. Our information network works more effectively. Communication between our brain and body improves. Our self—awareness reaches a higher level. Our body becomes sensitive.

A friend of mine once told his big discovery to me. He found that every time when he was under stress, he had diarrhea. This is understandable. When we are under stress, a certain portion of our body will become tense, and the portion varies from person to person. In his case, it was his digestive system. A part of body under a long period of tension will eventually develop a disease. What exactly is disease? Disease is dis—ease or not—ease. Comparing my friend's self—awareness level with people who had a disease and did not know what caused it, his self—awareness level is higher than them. But according to Tai—ji standards, his self—awareness level is still very poor, since he found the problem after the tension had developed into the disease. That is too late!

After practice of Tai—ji exercises, you will find that even before your tension develops further, you have already sensed the change. By relaxing the tension, you are free from many problems that you had before.

From the above discussions, we understand that through the pursuit of Tai-ji martial art skills, a person can develop a very high level of self-awareness which are the primary factors of physical and mental well-being. So at one time, I thought the only way to gain better health is to pursue in the martial art aspect of Tai-ji Quan. The martial art requirements are generally more strict. As your skill improves, your health improves as well. As time went by, and my understanding of Tai-ji became deeper, my thoughts changed. I applied Tai-ji principles to my running. My running improved. I went to learn ball-room dancing. With my Tai-ji fitness, neither Latin body motions nor Tango Walk is difficult for me to master. I played ping-pong. I found my ping-pong ball skill was even better than that when I was a teen-ager. I realized that as long as we understand Tai-ji principles and apply them to our activities, we will benefit.

Tai-ji fitness exercises introduced in this book were designed such that by working on efficiency, self-awareness, self-control ... we are able to benefit from this ancient Chinese wisdom without learning how to fight. Tai-ji fitness exercises can be practiced by anybody. You do not need to have any special talent. Tai-ji exercises bring you back to nature. Tai-ji exercises return you the things that nature offers you, the things with which we were born, but lost and forgot later in life.

The most important thing is that through the above discussions we now understand how and why millions people benefit from Tai-ji Quan practice in China. You can gain better health from wholistic or metaphysical approaches which can be found everywhere in the United States. In my opinion, Tai-ji approach is the easiest and the most beneficial way. Tai-ji training is a comprehensive physical and mental fitness exercise. It is a combination of metal approach and physical approach. It can be practiced anywhere. It is economic. Moreover, it is fun to do.

Fitness

The word "fitness" means different things to different people. To some, it means the ability to finish a workout exercise. To others, it may mean fitting into a smaller size dress. A person who is strong in weight lifting is not necessarily a fit person. So, what is Tai–ji fitness? I summarize the Tai–ji fitness as the following: According Tai–ji fitness principles, through the practice of Tai–ji Quan or Tai–ji exercises, to achieve the following results:

1. Being in balance in all aspects with a good flexibility and elasticity.
2. Being able to do everything efficiently.
3. Having a higher degree of self–awareness.
4. Having a higher degree of self–control.

There is a difference between fitness and sport. A person good in sport is generally very fit, but a very fit person may not be good in sport. One importance point is that a fit person may learn sport quickly. Another more important point is that a fit person may have a healthier body than a specific sport athlete, since over–all balance or total fitness is the key of health.

Many people gave up learning Tai–ji Quan because they do not understand the reasons. Many people practice Tai–ji Quan but make very poor progress because they do not get the essentials. Many people do not want to learn Tai–ji Quan because they are not interested in martial arts. In this book, I provide you a solution that is to practice Tai–ji fitness exercises and apply Tai–ji principles to your exercises. I hope my words here will help you to understand the reasons and reveal the mystery of Tai–ji Quan so that everybody can benefit from it.

Way of Tai-ji

Tai-ji training is precise and detailed. This is the way of Tai-ji. By and large, one takes a longer time to benefit from Tai-ji exercises. True logic is easy to say, but not so easy to actually apply to a tangible action. For example, the static stretching definitely gives the quickest approach to a large range of motion. Tai-ji stretching may take a longer time to get the same range of motion. But the quality will be different. Some Tai-ji exercises have to be practiced slowly. Therefore patience and concentration are required. This is the common difficulty many people, especially young people encounter in Tai-ji practice. However, once you experience the first benefit, and the difference in quality, you will enjoy the slow and gentle Tai-ji fitness approach.

The pursuit of preciseness results in good self-control. The pursuit of detail results in the total fitness. Therefore, we should not consider Tai-ji exercises too precise and too detailed. The uniqueness of Tai-ji lies in its preciseness and detail. If you practice Tai-ji training in a very rough manner, you will loose all the special benefits Tai-ji provides.

"No exercise can train a muscle for all of its possible functions. More important, no general exercise is as good as sport-specific performance." experts Richard Mangi, Peter Jokl and O. William Dayton said in their book "Sports Fitness and Training." They also said "If you want to be a better golfer, play golf !" I understand the above points, but do not agree totally with this theory. When people move, there are some things which are fundamental. Overlooking the fundamental skills will not allow us to advance further. The training introduced in this book deals with the fundamental skills. This is the Tai-ji approach.

What differentiates Tai-ji Quan from the other martial arts is not primarily from the martial art skills or its sport-specific skills. It is the basic training and its result, Tai-ji fitness, which differentiates Tai-ji Quan from the others. I personally believe that after a person achieves Tai–ji fitness, if he practices martial arts, he will be a good martial artist, if he plays golf, he will be a good golfer. Tai–ji fitness is a basic fitness.

How can a slow and soft styled Tai–ji Quan be considered as a martial art? Can it be effectively used in self–defense? This is a confusion among many martial arts fans. In fact, the Tai–ji Quan shadow boxing form is similar to Jane Fonda's low impact workout. It is a type of fitness exercises. To be a martial artist, you need to add the martial art specific skills to it. With the degree of the difficulty that Tai–ji requires, how can we practice it fast in the beginning? A fast beginning means overlooking specific details, and results in building a weak basis on which later more difficult movements will depend on. A strong foundation is essential.

I summarize the Tai–ji circular approach to fitness as follows:

Physical strength — *through slow circular resistive movements*
Coordination — *through slow and fast circular movements*
Flexibility — *through bigger circular movements*
Elasticity — *through fast circular movements*
Agility — *through fast and small circular movements*

In addition, we gain sensitivity through relaxation, gain self–awareness through the pursuit of efficiency, gain control through the pursuit of preciseness. We then are able to reach a state where we have super body, super self–control, super self–awareness, super sensitivity, and super efficiency. This is the "Tao" of Tai–ji.

3. BASIC EXTERNAL TRAINING

In each of the following sections, you will find clear instructions on how to practice each step with pictures and illustrations. If you follow the instructions and refer to the book as much as you need to, your body will learn these exercises and make them a natural part of your everyday life.

Tai—ji Quan is one of the internal martial arts in China. Therefore, many people are interested in its internal aspects such as "Qi" or "Chi". After reading this section, you will find that Tai—ji basic training is also very external. The requirements are rigorous and strict. The rewards are internal. You may be wondering that how long you need to learn the skills through the exercises. The answer is that is "depends". I can tell you that the skills described in this section took me 3 years to master them. Of course, I started practicing Tai—ji Quan at age of 25, and I have taken many detours. With the help of this book, your should see benefits in just a few weeks.

General Points

The following exercises are designed to improve muscle tone, increase flexibility, increase muscle strength, improve posture and promote a healthy energy flow in your body. Especially, the exercises are designed to improve coordination and efficiency of your movements. In addition, the exercises will coordinate body and mind and produce greater feelings of calm and grace. You should find that most of the exercises are fun to do.

Here are some basic rules:

1. Do it at a well—ventilated place.
2. Do it at least an hour after eating.
3. Wear loose—fitting clothes.
4. Do it gradually. Gently stress your natural capacity.
5. Never force yourself to do anything. Train not strain.
6. Exercise regularly. Be consistent.
7. Follow the Tai—ji principles.

Shaking

Starting with your head, shake each part of your body. After shaking your head, shake your shoulders, then arms, hands. waist, hips, followed by legs, ankles and feet.

The purpose is to loosen your entire body and get ready for other exercises. This exercise is best to do in the beginning of each practice.

Touching

This exercise will help you to relax your body and mind. It also develops your tactile sensation. It has a calming effect.

First, shake your hand and arms such that your fingers, hands and arms are totally relaxed. Then touch your body with your fingers, and move them slowly all over your whole body, from head to toes. Use one hand at a time. The touch should be light and gentle. As your fingers move, focus your entire attention on the feeling of touch. Based on my experiences, this exercise puts you quickly into the proper mood for Tai-ji exercises.

Body Checking

This exercise will help you become more sensitive to your body and allow you to relax thoroughly so that efficiency can be achieved. This is the basic step to achieve a sensitive body. The sensitivity of our body is the important step to achieve total relaxation. Total relaxation is the most important step to achieve efficiency.

Stand with feet shoulder width apart and knees slightly bent, review what occurs in your body. Do an inventory check of your body from your head down to your toes, asking yourself the following types of questions:

1) Is my breath deep?
2) What I can sense from this part of my body?
3) Is that part of my body relaxed?
4) Am I efficient and "sink" ?

When you first start to practice this exercise, you may try to start from your head skin, facial muscles, neck .... After you practice this exercise many times, you may gradually go to details, such as head skin, eyebrow, eyes, ears, lips, jaw, etc. In the beginning, this exercise may take you a long time to do. Eventually, this exercise should be done in a second or so. Get used to this type of mental exercise. Do not worry about what you can not sense. Put the parts you can sense onto your inventory list first and simply go through it. Learn to analyze yourself and make this as your habit. This exercise is required to practice through out all Tai-ji exercises. "Check you body" will be constantly referred to in the following exercises, meaning do this exercise.

Arm Rising and Falling

This exercise will help you become more sensitive to your arms and allow you to gain full control of your arms and gain a relaxed and alert upper body.

Stand with feet shoulder width apart and knees slightly bent. Check your body. Then raise your arms in front of you, hands are shoulder width apart, stop at shoulder height then drop them back to the sides of your thighs. As you raise your arms, initiate the movement from your shoulders, then elbows, wrists, finally hands, as you lower the arms, keep the same order, shoulders, elbows, wrists and hands. In the entire process, keep your arms relaxed, breathe naturally, do not pay attention to your breathing, make the arms move as slow as possible, no stop is allowed, for each rise or fall. Do it at least for 30 seconds, if you have no clock near by, count 30 for rise and 30 for fall. After you are able to do this exercise in 60 seconds with ease, then pay attention to evenness.

This arm movement is used in Tai-ji Quan commencing form. After I learned the simplified 24 forms Tai-ji Quan, I heard that the commencing form alone will need a full year to practice. At that time, I was really at a loss. I tried to believe the theory, but did not know where to put my effort. I am sure many of Tai-ji practitioners also share the same feeling with me, after having learned the forms, do not know where to go, how to further advance in the art. One of my purpose in this book is to provide some details so that you can learn the knack of Tai-ji Quan.

Why do we need to do this boring exercise? Because this exercise gives us relaxed, alert and full controlled arms. If you often cut your hands, or burn your hands, or drop things to ground while doing things in yard or at work, or break dishes while washing them, or sometimes have problem catching a ball in your favorite ball game. You should spend more time on this exercises seriously. Of course, if you practice martial arts, and have difficulty to do this exercise, I would not be surprised if you can not block a punch as you wish.

This exercise will make you do things with felicity. The following exercises may not always have the arms involved, but the relaxed arms gained from this exercise should always remain while you practice other exercises.

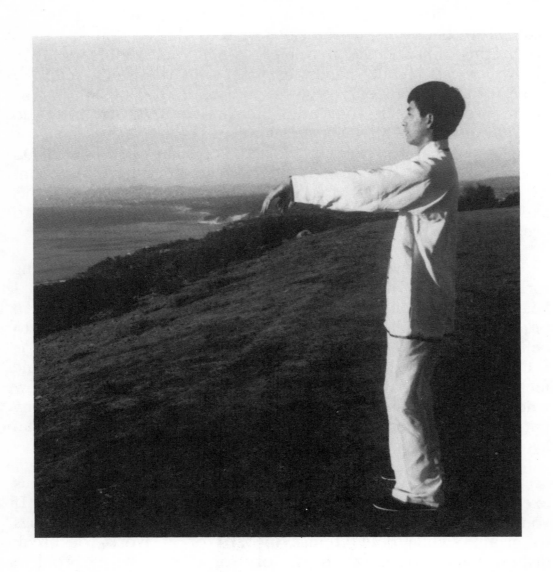

Hip Circling

The hips are the most important part of our body. Hip flexibility is very essential to many sports and daily activities. This exercise is called the hip circling exercise. Actually, it trains other parts of body as well.

Stand erect with two feet a little closer than shoulder width. Bend your knees slightly. Check your body, then draw a circle movement with your hip. Start from a small circle, and move slowly. Do not allow any abrupt move, make the circular movement as smooth and fluent as possible. Circle in both directions.

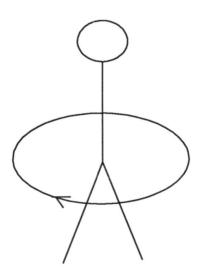

Figure 3-1 Hip Circling

Combine breathing into the exercise. Inhale in the front half circle, exhale in the rear half circle.

While practicing this exercise, you should have a feeling that each part of your body is grinding each other. The grinding makes your body, especially the joints, warm from the inside. It is the best way to tune-up your rusty joints and body. Static stretching gives pressure to certain portion of body. This tends to block the blood circulation in that portion of the body. Unlike the static stretching, the gentle circular motion provides a periodical stimulation to the body, the metabolism is therefore promoted so that aging in your bones and joints is reduced. The gentle circular grinding motion makes the cartilage change gradually, so that stiffness can be completely removed. The grinding also strengthens bones, joints and muscles so that the risk of exercise injury is reduced. You may feel cracks in your hip joints while making the moves. The first objective is to get rid of the cracks. Depending upon your age, it may take some time to develop flexible joints. Of course, if you are young, you do not have this problem.

Figure 8 Moving

Moving in a figure 8 pattern is essential to Tai-ji training. For convenience, let name the figure 8 patterns as shown in the Fig. 3-2. What is so important about a figure 8? Figure 8 has an interesting characteristic that it contains two circles. One is clockwise. The other is counterclockwise.

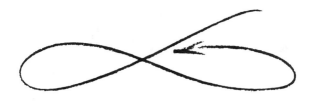

FORWARD FIGURE 8

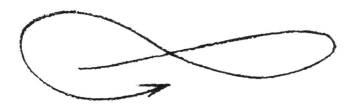

BACKWARD FIGURE 8

Figure 3-2 Figure 8 Patterns

As we move our body around, for example, from left to right, our body's movement basically interchanges between these two circles. Smoothly interchanging between these two circles gives us the ability to move our body quickly. If I say the circular movement is the first step to agility, then the figure 8 is the second step. If you happen to know wrestling, your technique and strategy lies in how good you move between the two circles. The art of grabbing and ungrabbing or parrying and attacking in self-defense lies in the art of clockwise circles, counterclockwise circles and smooth transitions. Therefore, when you practice this exercise, while making the two circles as round as possible, pay special attention to the transition between the two circles, make the transition as smooth as possible. The following exercises go gradually from easy to difficult. According to the situation, you may stop at any level.

Step 1: Imagine a center point between your hips, draw a figure 8 as shown in Fig. 3-2. Actually, as your center point is drawing a figure 8 pattern, your two hips are drawing circles respectively. As you draw the figure 8 patterns, your weight should shift between your balls and heels as shown in Fig. 3-3. As you shift to the right, relax your left body. As you shift to the left, relax your right body. Be efficient!

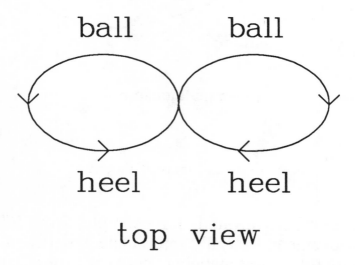

front

ball   ball

heel   heel

top view

Figure 3-3 Diagram of Weight Distribution

Step 2. Draw variation patterns as shown in Fig. 3–4. The curves are not continuous for illustration purposes. In practice, all the curves should be smoothly connected. These are two ways to interchange between the forward and the backward figure 8 patterns.

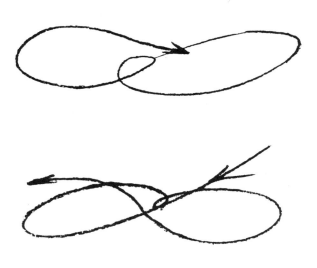

Figure 3–4 Pattern Variation 1

Step 3. Draw variation pattern 2 as shown in Fig. 3–5. These are two other ways of interchanging between the forward and the backward figure 8 patterns.

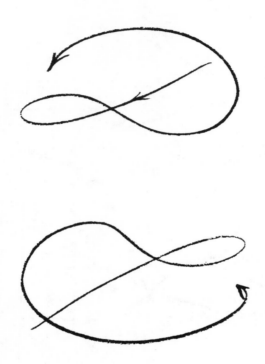

Figure 3–5   Pattern Variation 2

Step 4: Draw a combination of the patterns.

Step 5:   Change foot location from Fig. 3–6 to Fig. 3–7. Repeat the above exercises.

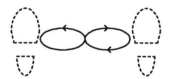

Figure 3–6   Foot Position 1

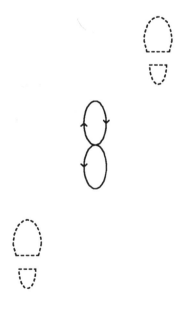

Figure 3–7   Foot Position 2

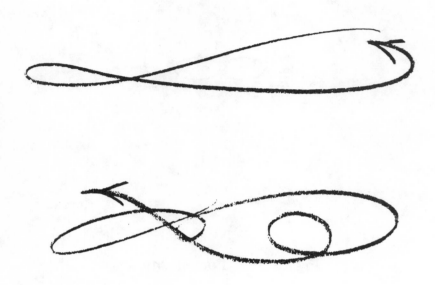

Figure 3–8 Pattern Variation 3

Step 6: Change the shape and the speed. Two examples are shown in Fig. 3–8.

Do not allow any discontinuity because it means loss of balance and control in applications. Speed does not need to be kept constant, but smoothness and evenness must always be kept. As you gain mastery, keep your body leveled. In other words, shift your body while moving at a constant level. In this way, the coordination of your legs will be proved.

54

Waist Twisting

This exercise trains the twisting strength of the spine. This movement is essential to many sports. When you practice this exercise, the key here is to promote the stretch reflex.

Draw figure 8 with twisted spine. Keep your body erect. Imagine your spine as a torsion spring, wind and unwind it back and forth. Fig. 3-9 shows the top view of your body movement, the unwind portion is where the stretch reflex plays its role. Let the arms swing freely. They will pat on your body. It is a massage to your body.

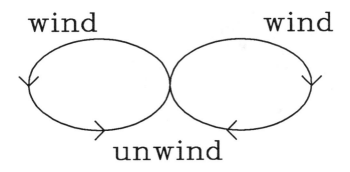

Figure 3-9 Spine Twisting Pattern

I do not play tennis very well. The first time I played with my friend, he was surprised to see that I handled the back stroke fairly well. He thought I had a talent for the sport. I did not say any thing. I tell you now, this is totally due to my Tai-ji fitness, especially the figure 8 shifting and the waist twisting training. I did not use my arm only, I used my whole body and initiated from the hip with a pre-wound spine (controlled stretch reflex).

The hip circling, the figure 8 moving and the waist twisting exercises are all working on the middle portion of your body. The massage effect to your lower abdomen will improve your reproductive and digestive functions. It is also an effective way to trim fat around your waist. Once this skill is mastered, the power of the hip increased. In Tai-ji Quan and many other sports, we need to use whipping type of force. That is to imagine the waist as a "handle" of a whip and the hand as tip of the whip. How effective you can use this whip depends very much upon how well you move the "handle". These three exercises are working on the "handle".

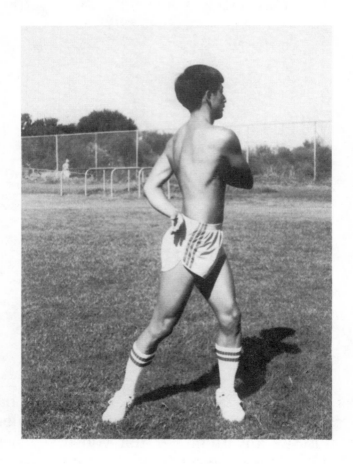

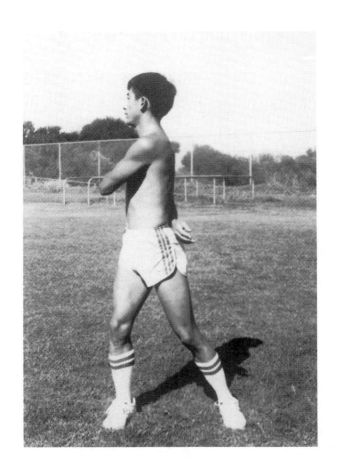

After you can practice this exercise fluently, keep your gravity center at a constant level. This demands a good correlation of legs. It will improve your leg coordination and in turn improve your skill and speed to shift your body's center of gravity.

Leg Stretching

Hips and knees are very important parts of your body. This exercises is mainly a hip and knee stretching exercise. It trains the flexibility of your legs.

Take a stance, an example is shown in the picture. Check your body. Draw circles with knees in all possible directions and combinations. Ankles and hips should be kept loose during the entire exercise. This is not only leg stretching exercise. The ankles and hips are also stretched.

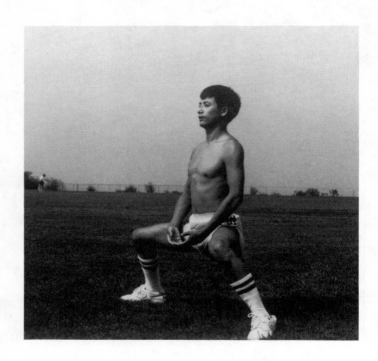

58

Gradually separate your feet further apart, and bend your knees further. This will strengthen your legs. This will improve the flexibility of your knees. As I described in the flexibility section, while you continue to separate your feet and lower your stance, it stretches your hips and legs in all-around directions.

To check your flexibility, bring your knee high in front, then pull the knee to your side. See if you can keep your knee at the same height as you pull your knee. For most people, as they pulled their knee to the side, the knee started to go down. This is because most stretching exercises train the forward direction. The hurdle stretch only trains the side direction. This exercise trains us in all-round flexibility. After you practice this exercise, you will be able to raise your knee forward high then pull your knee to your side without lowering your knee. Because this exercise stretches your muscles in circular motion, the muscles involved is strengthened. Elasticity of the muscles is improved. Therefore, this exercise provides us with a better resistance to hip and knee injury.

Knee Rolling

This exercise is aimed to develop leg coordination which is the most common difficulty people encounter in Tai-ji practice. Drawing circles requires a very good leg coordination. The importance of neutralizing coming force has been discussed in the section "Mechanics of Tai-ji". I will not discuss it here again. Mastery of circular movement is the key to have a fluent connection between different movements. In other words, It is the key to be agile.

Step 1: Take a stance. An example is shown in the picture below. Another example is the picture shown for the leg stretching exercise. Draw a vertical circle with your body. You may choose the stance you use in your sport. Be "sink" all the time!

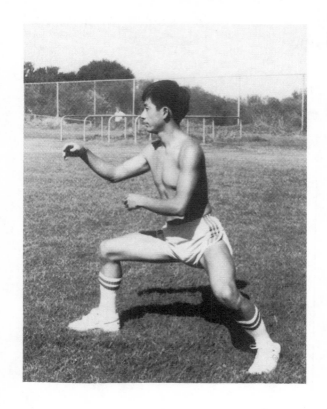

Step 2: Change the shape, keep the smoothness.

Step 3: Draw a vertical figure 8 as described in the previous exercise.

If you want to improve your agility and coordination, this is an effective exercise. Some people have strong legs, but can not deliver a powerful push. This is because when the rear leg extends, the front leg should bend, so that the total force is forward. With a poor coordination, the front leg can not bend in time. The two legs are fighting each other and most of the energy is wasted there.

Before my practice of Tai-ji, I had tried stair jumping, running and other knee related exercises. After the practice of Tai-ji, I found that I still had a great difficulty adjusting my stance on a fine scale. All the exercises I practiced before fail to lead me to Tai-ji standard. An American Tai-ji teacher once told me that "practicing Tai-ji will change one's wooden legs to rubber legs." This is a vivid analogy. If you practice static stretching, because of the suppression of the stretch reflex, you will probably get plaster legs rather than rubber legs. The rubber legs are true for people who have practiced in all high, medium and low forms of Tai-ji Quan. After a person practices the forms in different height, he will be able to change his muscle tension in all angles smoothly. In other words, he will be able to change his height to a very fine degree. A great Tai-ji master Tu-nan Wu who is over 100 years old and lives in Beijing, recalled his Tai-ji training in an article. He was forced to practice the form under high tables.

After practicing this exercise, I found that my knees become very flexible. I also noticed that I can jump and land on the ground very lightly. The physics is the follows: When my feet first touch the ground my feet and knees are very relaxed. It is like putting the end of a rope to the ground. After the full contact between my soles and the ground, I then smoothly and gradually tense up my muscles. My landing becomes very light. Any sudden change in the tension of the muscles will cause an impact to the ground in turn make a loud sound. After you gain the strength and the control from this exercise, you will be able to do it.

The jumping exercise is too rough. It does not care about the process or what happens in between. It emphasizes result rather than process. You start rashly then wait for landing. It trains you how to go up and does not care how you land. The weight lifting exercise only concentrates on the up–movement. The knee rolling exercise trains your strength and coordination. Because the smooth curvature requires a very good coordination of both legs, it is an excellent coordination exercise. It gives a very special tone to your leg muscles. You will be able to adjust your legs with any angle of bending to very fine degree. How can you achieve it? Do it very slowly and fluently.

A story about the great Tai–ji Master Sun Lu–tong (the founder of Sun style Tai–ji Quan) was told as follows. Once his neighbor came to his house and told him that he saw a ghost in early morning. Master Sun asked him what the ghost looks like. He said that the ghost was about two feet in height and ran out of his sight in a flash. Master Sun laughed and told him that it was he practicing squat running in early morning. If a person can walk in squat position, he should be considered to be in good condition. You may argue that your sport does not require strength and control in that position. You therefore do not need to practice at lower angles. This is a flexibility or adaptability problem. Do we need strength and control in the angles less than 90 degree? Normally, we do not. But when we lose our balance, for instance, slip on an icy road, we do need it. The flexibility, strength and control at lower angles may therefore save us from severe injury or possibly save our life. This is why when I watched the Olympic Games, I felt sorry for the skiers who lost their balance in the race. They believe in the slogan "If you want to be a better golfer, play golf! " and overlooked the importance of flexibility and basic training. Why Taijists emphasize the flexibility? They learned from their past experiences. To athletes, this may simply mean winning or losing. To Tai−ji ancestors, this meant life or death.

Though the hip circling exercise and the figure 8 moving exercise train horizontal circular movements, and the knee rolling exercise trains vertical circular movements, you should not be constrained by this. The final goal is to move your body in a circle of any shape and speed in three−dimensions.

Foot Rotating

Rotate your foot around the ankle, 8 times in each direction. As you rotate your foot down, bend your toes down as much as you can. As you rotate your foot up, raise your toes up as much as you can. In this way, both feet and ankles are stretched.

Ankle Tilting

This exercise is basically the isolation exercise for ankles. We all know that Tai-ji requires good relaxation. But to what degree and details? The following exercise is a good example.

Before you do the exercise, find a place where the ground has a slope (about 15 degree) and stand with one foot on the sloped ground. Keep a full contact between your sole and the ground, relax your ankle. You will be surprised to find that you can keep a good balance with the tilted ankle, you do not need to use any extra force to balance yourself. Rotate your body to all directions. The purpose of this exercise is to build up your confidence, to get rid of your fear, and eventually to get rid of stiff ankles.

Ankle tilting exercise: Less cushioned shoes are recommended to practice this exercise. Check your body as you practice. Walk very slowly, relax your hips, thighs, knees, ankles and feet. Initiate the move from your hip. From the time your heels touch the ground, to when your feet lift off the ground, keep your ankles relaxed. Imaging that your feet can freely rotate around your ankles as shown in Fig. 3-10 and Fig 3-11. If the ground leans on one side, still give a full and even contact between your foot and the ground, and distribute your weight evenly on the foot. Gradually increase your walking speed.

After you are able to do this on a smooth road, walk on a bumpy road. Practice until you can do it without thinking. As long as you walk, you can practice this exercise. It does not need place, uniform, equipments and special time. You may also apply this exercise to running. You will find that your running becomes more fun and enjoyable.

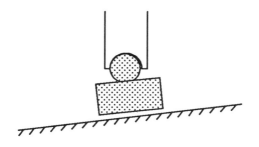

Figure 3-10   Rear View of Ankle Tilting

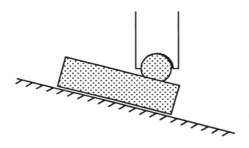

Figure 3-11   Side View of Ankle Tilting

What happens to most people is as the follows: When they walk on an un-level ground, because of their stiff ankles, the topology of the ground transfers to their shin bones. Since they can not evenly distribute their weight on their whole feet to keep balance with ankles tilted a little bit, the bumpy surface can not be isolated from the ankles bellow. They have to use force to counter-react in order to keep balance. What a hassle!

You may argue that relaxing your ankles will make your ankle sprained. If we do not move our ankles, our ankle muscles will not be strengthened. You are not asked to relax all the time. You are asked to relax in the beginning of each landing so that you can decide what to do. If the angle is within your flexibility, then you simply go on. If the angle is beyond your flexibility, then you do something else to avoid the sprain.

After you are able to walk with relaxed ankles without thinking, your balance will not be affected by the rough topology of the ground. You may then realize how miserable your old walk was. Moreover, this exercise improves the sensitivity of your feet and ankles.

I grew up in city and was spoiled by the industrial life. I assume most of you are not much different from me. For people who are gifted in sports or trained early in sports, this exercise and other exercises in this book probably should not be mentioned. Based on my experience, I was not alone, the majority of people share the same bad habits with me. Before I learned Tai−ji Quan, I was not much different from you. I had many bad habits and had great difficulty getting rid of them. This is why I have the following experience. I had found that all my shoes wore heavily on the outside edges. Before I learned Tai−ji, I thought that this was the way I was. It probably has been that way since I started to walk. It will never change. After I mastered the exercise described above, my shoes wear more evenly than before. I am able to walk on a bumpy road with ease. Recalling how many shoes I have worn with uneven wear, isn't that incredible? My ankle bones are still O.K. after all those years?

Toe Raising

A common phenomena is that after not using a specific part of the body for a long time, people lose control of that part. The headquarters (brain) has a poor communication with the part. The result is disease.

First, try to feel your big toe. Move it, and then the second and so on. You may have a problem doing it at first. After you are able to do this, stand up, shift your weight and feel the pressure change on your heel, ball and toes.

Step 1: Stand with feet shoulder width apart. Check your body, then gradually shift your weight from the heels to your balls, and from your balls to your toes. Do this back and forth.

Step 2: Stand on your big toes.

This exercise will enable you to balance yourself with the support from heel to toes. What commonly happens to people is that they mainly get support from heel to ball. This is good enough to do daily things. After doing this exercise, you will increase your toe strength. As a result, you will have better balance, because the base of heel–to–toe is wider than the base of heel–to–ball.

Note that this exercise increases toe strength, but does not ask you to tense your toes all the time, in contrary, you should relax them most of the time and tense them only when needed. Normally when people practice Tai–ji Quan, they learn the forms first. After mastering the forms, they then can concentrate on something else. For example, whether the hips are relaxed, the arms are relaxed. After all major body parts have been relaxed, they can pay attention to the details, such as whether the toes are relaxed or not. Many people have practiced Tai–ji Quan for years and have not reached the stage where toes and ankles can be considered. Training toes and ankles separately will speed up the learning time.

Tango Walk

When some people walk, they pound on the ground and make a loud noise. What really happen is that they have a habit of suddenly tensing their leg muscles when their leg lands on ground. Because their legs and knees are weak at certain angles. They do not allow their legs to bend further. They are afraid of loosing control. So they simply use extra force to suddenly stop the bending. Some people carry this habit to their running. There is no doubt they will have knee injuries. This habit creates great impacts to the knees.

Walk with bent knees, keep your body on a constant level. First put all your weight on one leg, and lift the other one forward. After the other foot lands on the ground, gradually shift your weight onto that leg. In order to keep the body leveled, the leg has to be stretched out at the landing, and gradually bent as the body moves onto it. When the total weight is on that leg, the leg bends the most. Walk in a figure 8 pattern, about 8 steps a circle, in this way, you are trained to walk curved in both directions. As you step out your front foot, point your toes to the direction you want to turn. A tension in your ankle and leg will be built. As you shift your weight on that foot, the stretch reflex will turn your body to the desired direction. Keep the feeling of "sink" all the time.

If you happen to know ball-room dancing, this walk is similar to the walk used in Tango. The goal is to eliminate the bad habit and get rid of the fear of letting your body further down. Bend your knees slightly in the beginning, gradually lower your body as you make progress. Combine this exercise with all other exercises previously described, you will gain good strength and control of your body. You will no longer fear the further dropping of your body. You can bring your body back up at any time and at any height. If your body goes down more, it will bounce back more. You will feel that you are a part of the earth, you are in harmony with the earth. This is the so-called "ground" or "rooting".

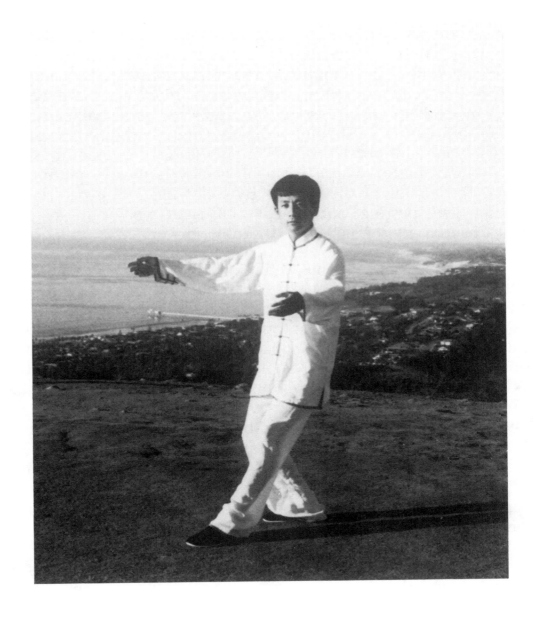

Rooting

Rooting or grounding are the terminologies by which Tai–ji practitioners refer to body movements or positions that are coordinated, balanced, controlled and efficient. All the exercises up to now are concentrated on this aspect. We all are born to walk. Because of the poor fitness of lower body, few of us walk lightly or move our body swiftly. In general, most of us tend to use more strength than what we really need, instead of using extra strength to gain balance and nimble moves, we should working on flexibility, control, coordination and efficiency. The world is designed in such way that no matter where we are, gravity is always pulling us toward the center of the earth. By following Tai–ji principles, relaxing and putting our body in a right position, we will always have a good balance and nimble movements.

Let me use an example, standing, to summarize what you have learned so far and what you should expect. Stand with feet shoulder width apart. Your feet should be relaxed. Your soles should follow the contour of the ground. Your toes should be relaxed and alert (ready to use force whenever it is needed). This is learned from the toe raising exercise. Your ankles should be relaxed. This is learned from the ankle titling exercise. If the ground is not leveled, your ankles are titled. Your knees should be bent. If the ground is not leveled, your knees should bend at different angle so that your center of gravity is centered. This is learned from the knee rolling exercise. You should use the minimum effort to support your weight. This is so–called "sink". This is learned from many exercises, especially from the Tango walk exercise. Your groin should be relaxed. This is learned from leg stretching exercise. Your hips should be relaxed. This is learned from the hip circling exercise. Your upper body should be relaxed. This is learned from the waist twisting exercise. Your arms should be relaxed. This is learned from the arm raising and falling exercise. If you can do all of this, you are "rooted". In other words, accept what is in front of you without wanting the situation to be other than it is. You are in harmony with the earth.

A student of mine once mentioned to me many good things swimming provides. He pointed out that there is no knee injury in swimming. I agreed with him totally. I like swimming myself. When I was in graduate school, I swam 3-4 times a week. But there is a hard fact we humanbeings have to confront. We have to use our legs to move our body around. The first aging sign in many old people is their knees. Therefore, we need to exercise our lower body in order to be younger and more productive in our daily work. Though a fit lower body does not seem to be as attractive and impressive as a strong upper body.

You probably have noticed that all the exercises are done in standing positions. I agree that relaxation exercises are easier to do in lying position. However, no matter how relaxed you are while lying on the floor, once you stand up, your body becomes tense again. As you start to move, the tension gets worse. Therefore, most of Tai-ji exercises are in standing positions.

If you happen to commute by bus or train, you may try the following interesting exercise. When you get on the bus, you may try to stand there without holding hangers. I am not going to tell you how to do it. Following the principles, you should have no difficulty to handle the normal stop, acceleration, and turn of the bus. Please try it. I guarantee that it is fun.

After the mastery of the skills introduced, you will find that, you can make a fake move in basketball or soccer easily and fast. You will become very slippery in Tai-ji push hand exercise. You will be able to shift your body and change your direction quickly. People in tennis talk about foot work. It really should be body work, or center of gravity work. Work hard on it and you will find the differences.

Walking Exercise

Have you noticed that some people do not walk, they waddle. After the basic external exercises are learned, you will find a change in the way you walk and the way you move your body. The joy can be described as a change from an economy car to a Cadillac. You get more horse power, better control, and a better suspension. Most of us do not have a Cadillac to drive. But now you have a "cadillac" to ride and it brings you anywhere. Wouldn't that be wonderful thing to have? Besides following the principles, here are some tips to make your walk more pleasant.

1. When you walk, do not stroll or shuffle. Instead move at a steady pace.
2. Hold your head erect as if suspended by a thread from above.
3. Toes point ahead
4. Concentrate on your walk.
5. Your arms should swing freely as they hang from your shoulders.
6. Breathe deeply.

Your brisk walk will then be admired by others. The Tai–ji classic treatise describes the way that Tai–ji practitioners walk as "while making a stride, it is as quiet and as light as a cat walks." If you are over–weight, walking will reduce your weight. If you are under–weight, walking will help you gain weight. The key is to keep it relaxed and rhythmic, and not less than 30 minutes. The external harmonic movement will stimulate your internal metabolism in such way that a metabolism balance is obtained.

Walking with weights is not recommended. It is clumsy externally so that your internal system is crippled as well. Tension in your body blocks your internal energy flow. A balanced metabolism can not be maintained and rehabilitated.

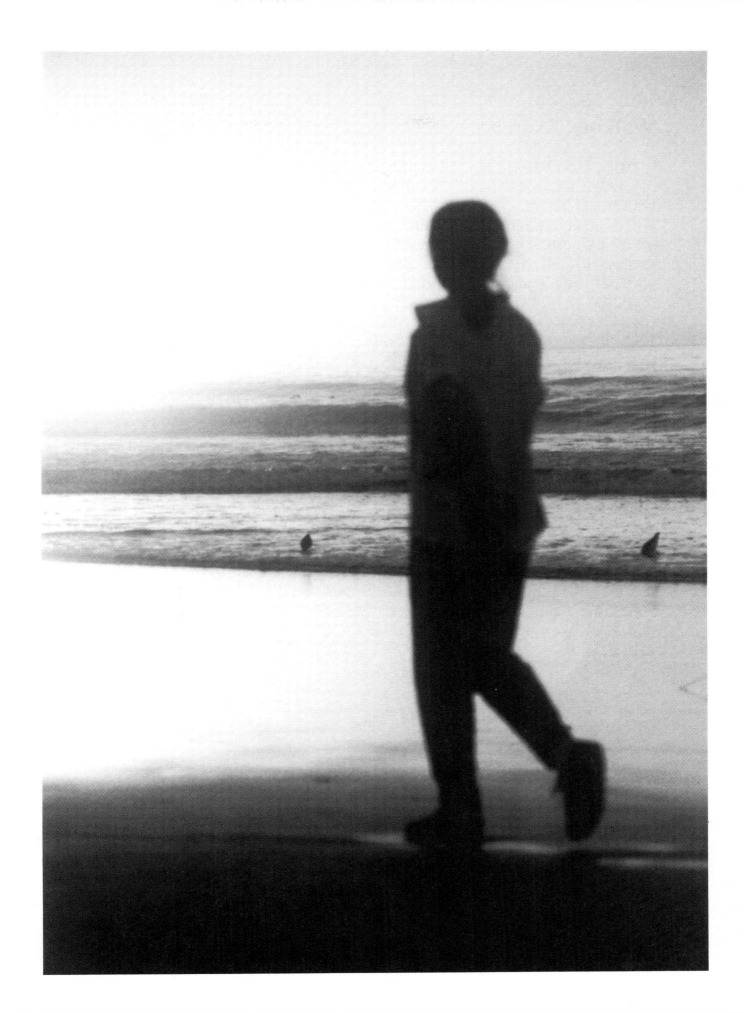

Spine Rocking

This exercise uses hand's circle motion to induce a wave-like movement of the spine as a fish does. In general, I agree with all the points of chiropractor. Therefore I assume you all understand the importance of healthy spine.

Exercise 1:   Stand with your knees bent, and raise your both hands in front, draw a circle as shown in Fig. 3–12 and the pictures.   While your hands reach out, bend your spine as the dotted line shown in the figure.   While pull your hands back, arch back your spine as the solid line.   Do it gradually and slowly.   Be relaxed.   You should feel every part of your body grinding each other.

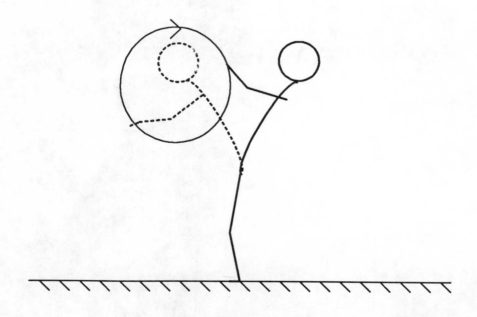

Figure 3–12 Spine Rocking Exercise

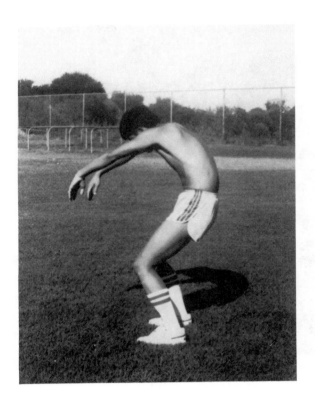

b.

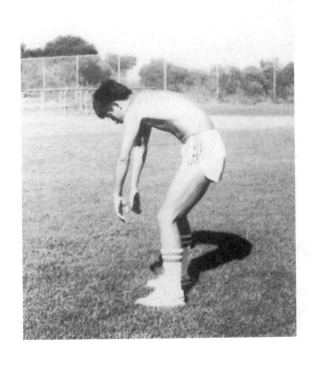

a.

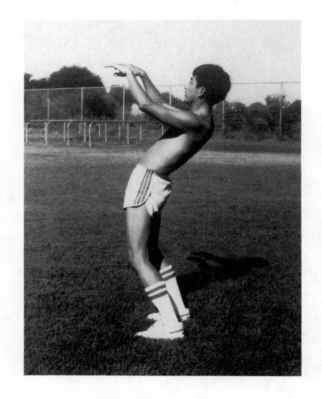

c.

d.

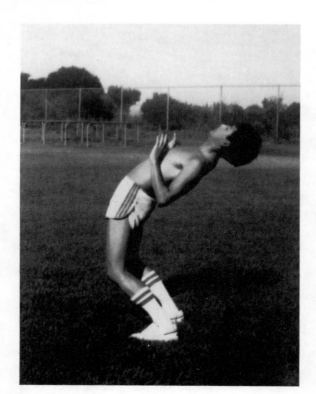

76

Exercise 2: Turn your palm toward you, fingers point to the sides and 2 to 3 inches apart. Draw the circle in the reverse direction.

Many spine exercises are practiced in a static fashion. The range of motion is emphasized, but the elasticity is overlooked. In this exercise, not only spine flexibility is trained, but also the bones and the muscles along the spine are strengthened. Resistance to back injury is therefore increased. Please do this exercise very gently. For many people, they have not stretched their back for years. If the exercise is done severely, injury may occur.

In the beginning, you may move your arms and spine only, then gradually add your lower spine, neck, shoulders, legs, knees and ankles into the movement. You may experience your body get warm quickly. You may also sweat a lot, but you will find that this sweat is different from the sweat you get from running or rope jumping. This is a wonderful exercise to attain balanced energy flow in your body. Your whole body moves in a rhythmic fashion. When you do static stretching, certain portion of your body is pressed such that blood circulation is blocked. When you do circular movements or waving movements, it stimulates your body periodically, so that your energy flow or metabolism is promoted. This is why Tai-ji has a wonderful healing effect. When the metabolism is balanced, a healthy body is achieved.

To move the lower portion of spine is easy. To move the center portion of spine is relatively difficult. To move the upper portion of spine is difficult. After you mastered the above exercise, you then can experience correct Tai-ji posture. Many other martial art styles use a posture as shown in Fig. 3-13. This posture is not efficient in asserting a force forward. The correct Tai-ji posture is shown in Fig. 3-14.

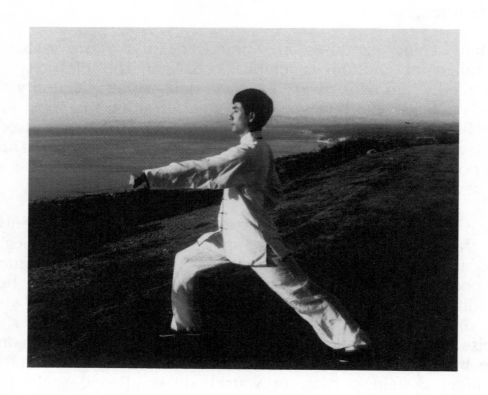

Figure 3-13 Incorrect Posture

After I was able to move my upper spine, my hunched back was corrected. Beauty is not the main goal of Tai-ji practice, but it is certainly a by-product of the exercise. After you are able to spring your spine like a fish trying to get rid of a hook, your body will become springy and powerful. For example, you will be able to have a strong tennis overhead serve or to do a strong and powerful spike in volleyball.

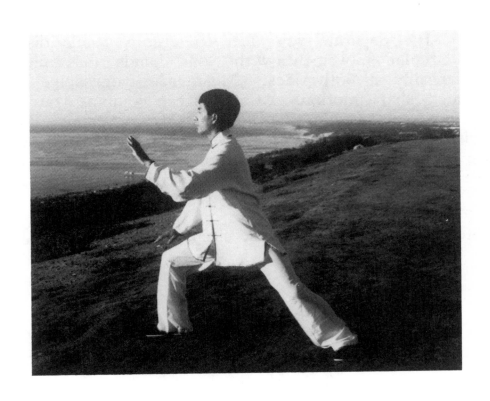

Figure 3-14 Tai-ji Posture

Side Reaching

The spine rocking exercise trains the spine flexibility in the front and back direction. This exercise trains the spine moving in the side direction.

Step 1: Separate your feet to a comfortable distance. Make circular movement with your hands (see pictures) interchangably at both sides. Meanwhile, your spine should make an S shape motion. After you can combine your upper body movements with your lower body movements in this exercise, you should find that your groin moves in a vertical figure 8 pattern. Do it in a relaxed manner. Do it as if you try to reach something on the side or as if you try to catch a ball.

Step 2: Do it in the reverse circular motion.

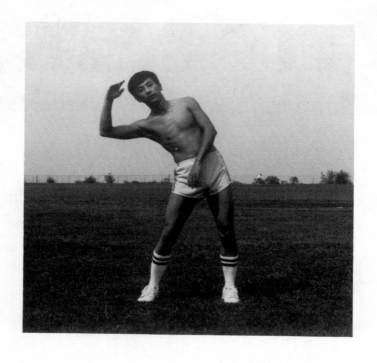

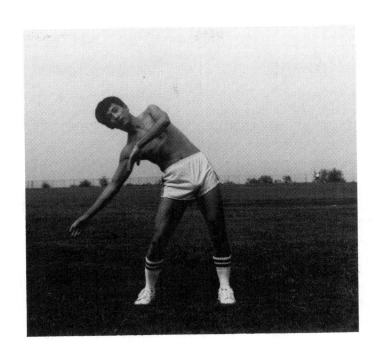

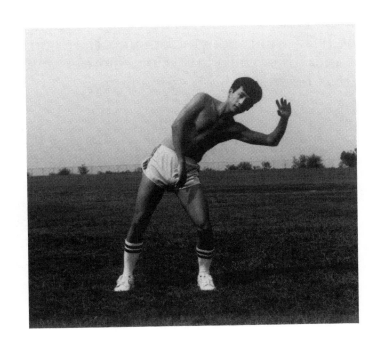

Shoulder Rowing

This exercise is primarily for increase of the shoulder flexibility and range of motion. The spine is also exercised. This is a good warm–up exercise. You should find that it makes you comfortable. Your body becomes warm from inside. As you practice the exercise, you should feel each part of your body is grinding each other.

Step 1: Relax your arms as they hang from your shoulders (picture a). Circle the right shoulder toward left, then up to the position shown in picture b.

Step 2: Continue circling the right shoulder to the position shown in picture c.

Step 3: Continue circling, and turn your left shoulder to the front.

Step 4: Circling the left shoulder in the natural opposite direction. Check your body. Combine the figure 8 motion of your hips and the waist twisting motion into it. Do it interchangably between both shoulders. Do it slowly and gently.

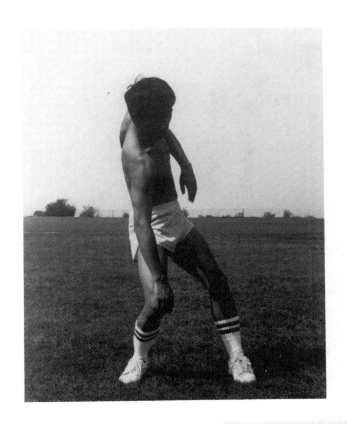

a.

b.

c.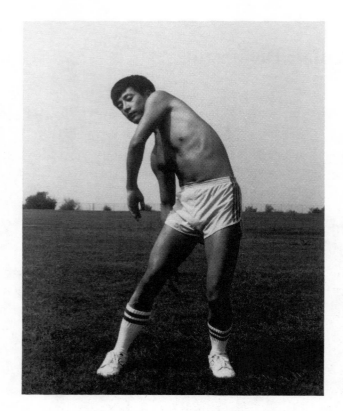

d.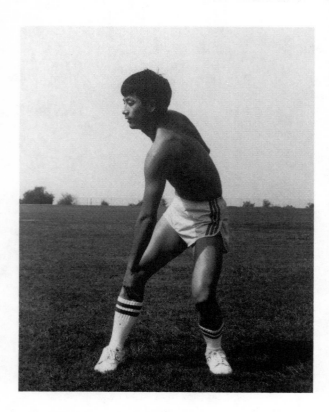

84

Circular Push-up

This exercise improves strength and flexibility of your arms and shoulders. The thing to remember is that weight training through a short range of motion will decrease flexibility. But, if you train through the entire range of motion of your joints, you actually increase your strength and flexibility.

Take a prone position, face to the ground, hands under shoulders and feet no more that one foot apart. Bring your hands and feet closer, so that when your arms and legs are straight, your body forms a triangle as shown in the picture a. Do this circular push-up exercise. When your body is in the up position, continue to raise your spine, so that the shoulder blades are in. When your body is in down position, continue to lower your chest, such that your shoulder blades are out. Inhale while raising your body, exhale while lowering your body. Think about how a cat walks, the shoulders are very relaxed, and the shoulder blades stand out.

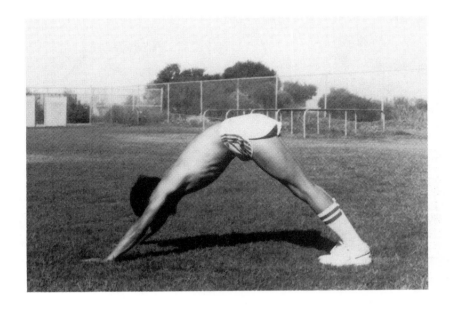

a.

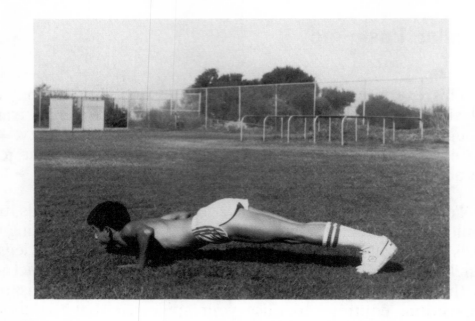

b.

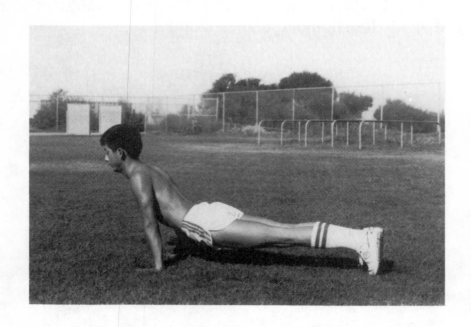

c.

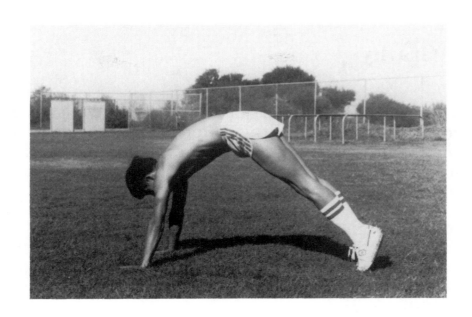

d.

This exercise is strength oriented. I have noticed that people pay attention to build big biceps. There is nothing wrong about it. But training of the shoulder muscles should not be neglected. Using biceps rather than shoulder muscles for some strength required movements is a bad habit, because it is not efficient and effective.

Let me tell you an interesting practice that uses Tai-ji principles. To open a tight glass container's cover is a typical problem we often run into. The way a person generally does is to open the cover by twisting the cover with wrist and forearm muscles only. Preferably, you should arch your shoulder forward, hold the cover with your hand, keep your wrist rigid. Use your shoulder and back muscles, stretch backward and pull the bottle slightly closer to your body. You should find that this gives a much easier way to open the cover.

This is only one example applying Tai-ji principles to daily life. I hope after reading this book you will apply Tai-ji principles to your daily activity and your favorite sport. Invent you own practice.

Use of Gravity

Efficiency is one of Tai-ji's essentials. We should do every movement with the least effort. It is impossible to cover all the details of each exercises. In this section, I introduce two exercises aimed at invoking your interest so that this principle can be applied generally.

Arm Swinging: Raise your right arm horizontally (Fig. 3-15). Move it to the left side. There are many ways to do this. Learn to relax your shoulder, let the arm swing to the other side. When the arm reaches the highest point, try to add very little force to have it stop there for a second before it swings back. This exercise teaches you to be efficient. Let the gravity to do the work.

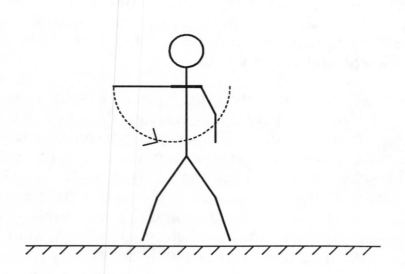

Figure 3-15 Arm Swinging

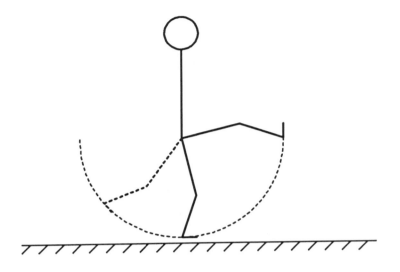

Figure 3-16 Leg Swinging

Leg Swinging: Lift one of your legs forward as high as you can. Hold in this position for a second then quickly relax all the muscles involved, especially the hip muscle. Let the leg swing freely to the dotted line position as shown in Fig. 3-16. Continue the motion of the backward moving leg. Gradually bring your leg upward as high as you can, then quickly relax your muscles and allow the leg swing forward. Do not stop the motion. Gradually tense your muscles and bring the leg as high as you can. You now are back to the beginning.   Do this repetitively, smoothly and slowly first. Once you are able to execute this exercise as the curve A shown in Fig. 2-5, you may increase the frequency of the exercise.

Running is one of my favorite sports. The above exercise is designed primarily for running. After you master this exercise, your muscle relaxation time will be improved. You may then test your skill in your running. If you can implement this skill in your running, namely, following the curve A in your running, you should find that your running becomes easier, faster and more enjoyable.

If you exercise regularly, you may say that "Ah I can do this, I just did not pay attention to this before." In this case, I first congratulate you for being fit. Then let us analyze the following case.

A person who is in poor physical condition, he will be using the curve C in running, after the running, his muscles will still be tense and sore for several days, this means that the muscle tension is still there, until the soreness goes away, his tension will go away finally. For a well-trained person, the tension and relaxation process is carried out between each stride in running. The difference in the relaxation time is between orders of magnitudes. This example gives us an idea how much difference we can create through exercises. This also tells us that the pursuit in dynamic efficiency is unlimited.

4. BASIC INTERNAL TRAINING

"Tai-ji Quan aims primarily at exercising our internal organs." said an expert of Tai-ji Quan. This is indeed true. This is why Tai-ji Quan is considered as an internal martial art. The substantial content of Tai-ji Quan's internal aspect is so profound and rich, that it is beyond the scope of this book. In this section, you will be exposed to the basic concept of Tai-ji internal training and some of the basic techniques I have developed.

Abdomen Moving

One time I mentioned to a student of mine internal muscle training.   He did a sit-up exercise, and asked "Is this what you mean?"   I replied "No".   The exercises in this section are the basic Tai-ji internal exercises.

Lie down with your face up in a comfortable place with bent knees.   Have somebody use their fingers to press into your stomach or you do this yourself.   Push out the fingers by using your internal muscles.   Practice at different portion of your stomach until you can push out the pressing fingers regardless of where they come from.   In the beginning, you may have to use your stomach as whole in order to push out the pressing fingers.   As you make progress, you will find that you can use localized muscles to push the pressing fingers out.   In other words, you are able to separate or isolate your internal muscles and control them individually.

The first phase of this exercise is to increase self-awareness of your internal organs, since you have to know where the fingers come from.   The second phase is to increase your internal muscle strength and flexibility, since you have to learn to push the pressing fingers out.   The third phase is to increase the efficiency and the control of your internal muscles, since you have to learn to use localized muscles to push the fingers out.   Finally, you may try to move your internal organs by yourself.   You should be able to move your internal organs according to your will.   At this stage, you have learned this basic skill.

Pay special attention to the lower abdomen.   The immediate goal is to stretch your abdominal muscle so that your internal organs can go down further.   Your diaphragm will be able to go down further.   As a consequence, Your vital capacity will be increased.   Your center of gravity can be further lowered, so you can gain a better balance.   The goals of this exercise are summarized as the follows:

1. *Increase self−awareness of internal organs*
2. *Increase self−control of internal organs*
3. *Increase internal muscle strength*
4. *Increase vital capacity*
5. *Increase flexibility of internal organs*
6. *Increase efficiency of internal organs.*

You may run a couple of miles a day or swim a couple of miles a day. Without specific training, you can not gain the vital capacity to its full extent. By practicing the Tai−ji breathing exercise under good guidance, you may eventually learn the above skill. This exercise enables you to learn it in a short period of time. As matter of fact, some people who practice Tai−ji Quan for many years still can not move their internal organs.

Practicing this exercise, your internal self−awareness and internal self−control will be improved. This is the prerequisite of internal efficiency. You may notice one thing after Tai−ji internal training. Your endurance and tolerance improved significantly. Part of the reasons is the improvement of your internal efficiency.

This exercise also keeps you away from many common diseases. Within few weeks of practice, problems such as constipation and diarrhea may go away. Medicine may no longer be needed. Also, having control of internal organs simply prevent us from suffering many common problems, for example, stitch. If the stitch is due to abdominal or intercostal muscle cramps, you may simply move the portion of your internal organs where you feel pain. At first it is hard to be moved, once it is moved, the stitch is gone.

Another interesting example is to stop hiccups. I will not tell you how to do it here. But I can tell you that after you practice Tai−ji exercises for a period of time, you will be able to do it. You will also experience a lot of changes happening in your body. I leave those for you to find out.

This exercise is one of basic internal muscle strength training. Talking about the internal muscle strength, a story is told as the follows: Master Yang Lu-chan (the founder of Yang style Tai-ji Quan) was once challenged by a big and strong challenger. To decline the challenge humbly, he suggested that his challenger punch into his stomach three times. If he moves a step or falls, he will admit defeat. The first two punches did not make him move at all. Angry by Master Yang's nonchalance, the third punch came even more vigorously. It was neutralized and recoiled back, sending the challenger back over 10 feet away.

In the later years of Master Yang's eldest son, he often locked himself in his room, and practiced Tai-ji meditation and breathing exercises. He laid on his bed and put one grain of rice on his stomach. With a "Ha" sound, the grain was shot up to the ceiling. These stories give us an idea how far we can pursue in the internal training.

Our abdominal cavity is not well protected, the organs within are vulnerable to direct injury. This exercise is also a good exercise for sport injury prevention. If your sport involves a lot of body contact, you may practice this exercise. It will increase the resistance to a blow to your stomach.

Breathing

Proper breathing energizes and fortifies the body, aids our thinking process, increases endurance and stamina, strengthens immunity to disease and adaptability to environment. In spite of the importance of breathing, few of us do it properly. Just as with the natural processes, deep breathing is something that children do automatically but that most adults have forgotten. Most people seem almost incapable of doing it correctly.

There are two basic features to proper breathing: depth and evenness. Most of us take shallow breaths, breathing from the chest only. This does not bring enough oxygen into to our body. Deep breathing also increases the flexibility of our internal organs and our rib cage. As we make our breath deeper, we also increase the range of motion of our internal organs, and strengthen our internal muscles. So in Tai–ji breathing exercise, deep breathing is required. You may wonder why evenness is important. Evenness requires good control over our internal muscles. As we pursue evenness of breathing, our internal muscle control is improved.

The basic Tai–ji breathing consists of two techniques. They are natural breathing and reversal breathing

Natural breathing: While inhaling, you expand the abdomen; while exhaling, you contract the abdomen.

Reversal breathing: The lower abdomen contracts as you inhale, and expands as you exhale. In other words, the diaphragm rises as you breathe in, and drops as you breathe out.

You can practice the breathing exercise in sitting, supine, lying or standing position. The keys are 1) gradually deepen your breath, and 2) after you are able to breathe deeply then pay attention to evenness.

If you walk regularly, you may practice the breathing exercises with your walking exercise. Breathing should be coordinated with the steps. The principle is to take the same number of steps for each inhalation or exhalation; gradually increase the number of steps taken – from two steps for each inhalation or exhalation up to nine steps for each inhalation or exhalation. Everybody knows that before any sport activity we should do some stretching in order to reduce possibility of injury. Do you know that deep breathing is a simple form of internal muscle stretching? So before exercise, gentle and deep breathing should always practiced together with regular stretching.

The reversal breathing technique is hard to learn. Here is an exercise to help you to learn this technique:

Stand with feet shoulder width apart, as shown in the picture, check your body, as you breath in, raise your body and raise your arms, meanwhile raise your internal organs as if they are brought up by your hands; As you breath out lower your body by bending your knees, meanwhile drop your internal organs as if your hands push your internal organs to your lower abdomen.

The basic external training is elementary school level. The internal training and the breathing exercises introduced in this section is middle school level. After mastery of the breathing and the internal exercises, my fitness improvement made a leap. My body changed completely. The joy can not be dreamed of before, since the joy can not be understood by people who have no such experiences.

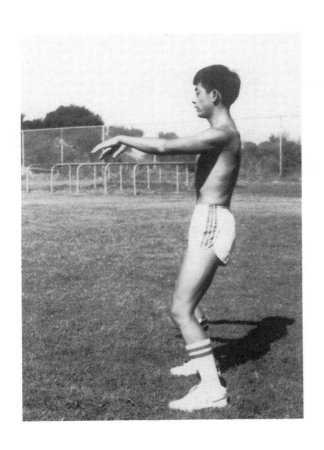

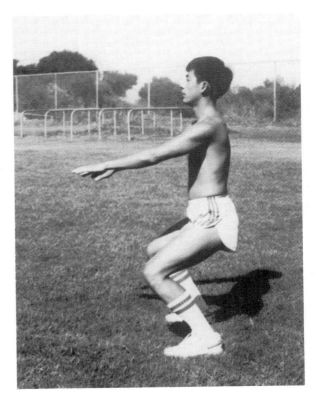

Back Breathing

I have talked to many people and asked them to do a deep breathing. What I observed is that they all have a great front rib expansion. But the spine is stiff, the rear ribs almost do not expand at all. This can be very easily understood. Laying on your back in a chair or sofa unable ourself to expand our spine and ribs backward. Therefore, the back breathing exercise is a little bit difficult. The next exercise will assist you to do the back breathing correctly.

Back breathing exercise: After the spine rocking exercise is mastered, you can then practice the back breathing exercise.

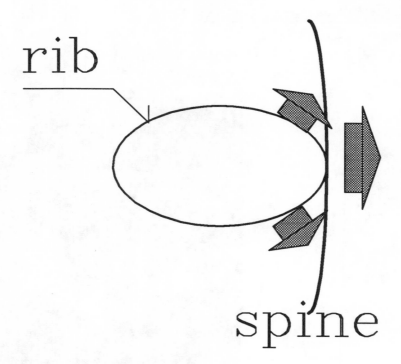

Figure 4-1 Back Breathing Illustration Chart

98

Cross your arms in front your chest and put your hands on the opposite shoulders (see pictures). Practice the reverse breathing, and expand your rear ribs gently. When breathing in, you should arch the upper spine backward. Meanwhile try to use the upper spine's outward going movement to lead the expansion of rear ribs (see Fig. 4-1). This will give additional room for your lungs. Do the deep breathing 4 repetitions a set.

People who practice Tai-ji Quan must have learned the two classic principles about the upper body posture. The direct translation has been the follows:

1. "Hollowing the chest" (Han-xuong)
2. "Lifting the back" (Ba-bei)

I have read from an article in a Chinese Wu-shu magazine. The article pointed out that the above two requirements are basically one thing. That means if one is done correctly the other is done correctly as well. Besides this article, I have not found a satisfactory explanation.

Recently, in a Chinese Wu-shu magazine, there is even a debate about the two principles because some people taught the principles as keeping the shoulders slightly forward. They argue that these two principle give an unhealthy posture. They think that the two principles ask people to have a hunchback like a weak old man. I now would like to use this chance to clarify the confusion and give credit to our Tai-ji ancestors.

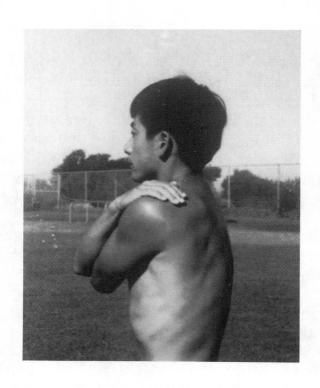

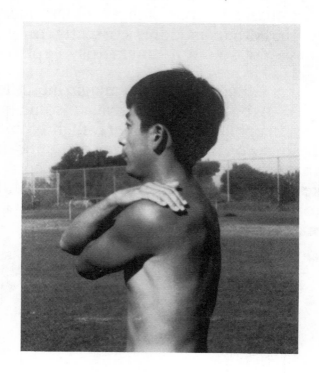

What the two principles mean, according to my understanding, is to use full thorax breathing with emphasis on the back breathing as we just discussed. "Lifting the back" means to use the back breathing. The bowing of the spine gives a sort of feeling that you lift your back. "Hollowing the chest" means to relax the chest. When the spine goes backward and your rear ribs expand, your shoulders with respect to your spine are truly slightly forward as some people teach. The point is that without the backward expanding of the spine and the ribs, bending the shoulder forward will definitely form an unhealthy posture. The goal is to breathe deeply without expanding the chest too much, such that chest muscles remain relaxed. In this way, the reaction time and the agility of arms will not be affected by breathing.

Because of the difficulty in arching the spine backward, most people who practice Tai-ji do not even get a feel of it. According to the traditional teaching system, the two principles can only be mastered through Tai-ji breathing exercise which is taught by few Westerners. I hope this discussion will clarify the confusion and bring prosperity to the learning of Tai-ji fans. In addition, I hope to bring health and excellence to the total fitness of exercising people. As far as I am concerned, this is the best, the healthiest principle or technique in the world. I would like leave the further discussion to sport and medical experts.

You should find that after the practice of this exercise your back muscles become much more relaxed and sensitive. Many people suffer back pain. Because, they tense their back muscles without knowing it. This exercise teaches you how to be free from such problems.

Rib Expanding

The rib expanding exercises are introduced as breathing exercises in Tai–ji school and many other forms of traditional Chinese fitness exercises. The exercises are done with very simple arm movements. Because a major effect of these exercises, rib expansion is not pointed out, many people are not interested in them. Therefore, I introduce the following exercises as rib expanding exercises, since this is the essential of the exercises.

Many people do not pay enough attention to the breathing exercises. In fact, they are the most important part of Tai–ji internal training. The following breathing exercise set is the basic standing form.

The breathing can be either natural or reversal in this exercise. If you choose to do the natural breathing, complete the whole set, then you may start another set using the reversal breathing. Do not mix the two. Make sure your stomach is in and out for each breath. To increase your internal organ flexibility and increase your internal muscle strength, breathing with the commencing posture is good enough. The next 5 exercises provide additional benefits. They are the flexibility of your rib cage and strength of muscles around your rib cage.

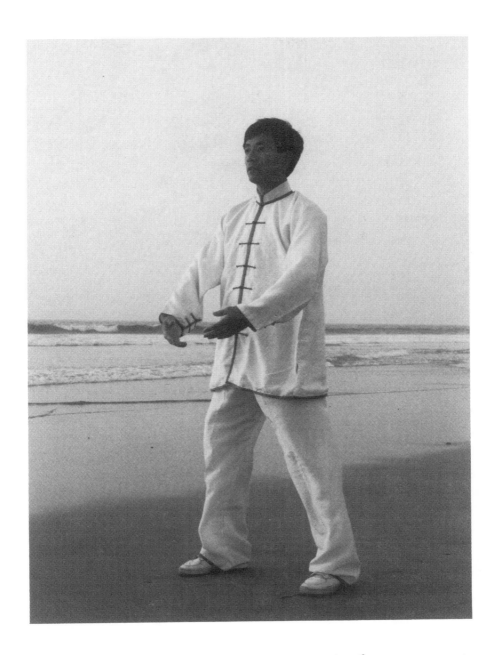

Commencing form: Hold your arms in front your stomach as shown in the picture, feet shoulder width apart, your arms and hands form a circle as if clutching a large ball, hands are about 3 inches apart, palms face your body. Check your body. Be "sink". Place tip of your tongue lightly against roof of your mouth and breathe through your nose. Breathe deeply 4 times a set. The following exercises should follow the same rules.

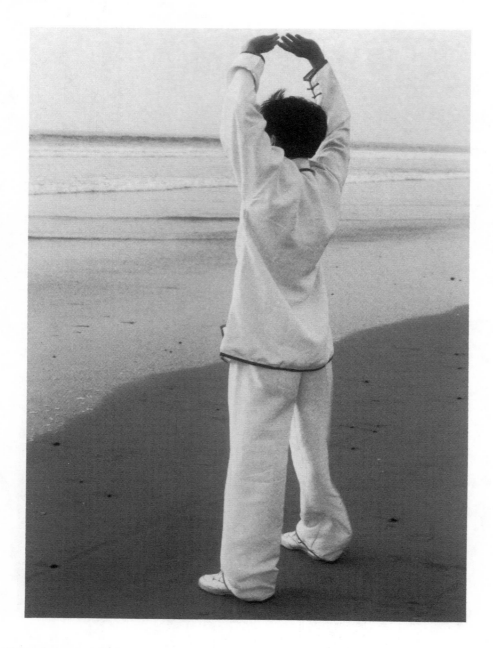

Chest expanding exercise: Breathe in slowly, as the same time, raise your arms over your head (see picture), keep your posture erect, in the entire process, your body should be relaxed. As you breathe in, besides the movement of your diaphragm, your rib cage should also expand. This exercise emphasizes the chest expansion. Breathe out, relax your body, drop your arms back to the commencing form.

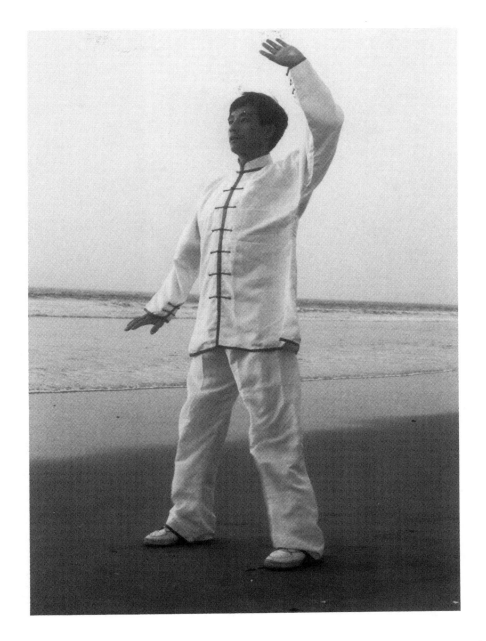

Side rib expanding exercise: Breathe in slowly, meanwhile, turn your left palm down and press your palm downward, turn your right palm to front then above, raise your right arm to the posture shown in the picture. As you raise your right arm, stretch the right side of your rib cage. You should focus to the feeling of your side rib expansion. Breathe out, relax your whole body, bring your arms back to the commencing form. Do the natural opposite of the above exercise.

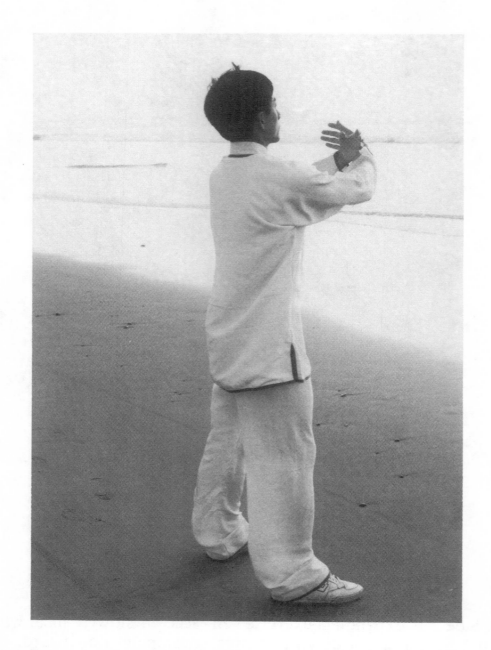

Back rib expanding exercise: Breathe in slowly, raise your hands in front of you to your shoulder height, form a cross as shown in the picture. This exercise mainly stretches your back. Breathe out, relax your body, drop your arms back to the commencing form.

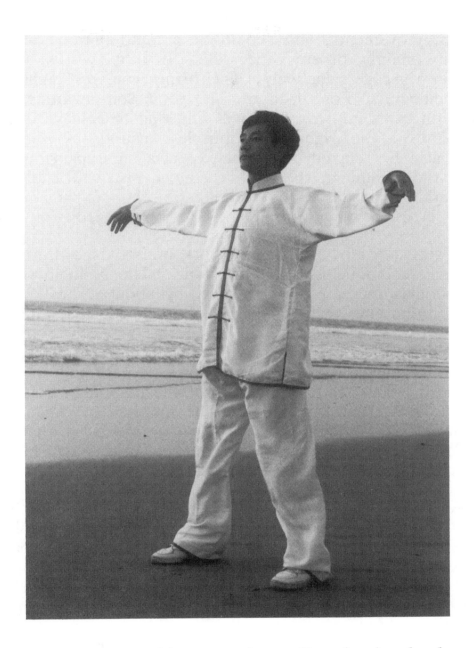

Full thorax stretching exercise: Breathe in slowly, raise your arms to the side at shoulder height. This exercise stretches your rib cage in all directions. Breathe out, relax, bring your arms back to the commencing form.

After you master these techniques, without the help from the arm movements, you should be able to breathe with the right ribs mainly, or any other side. In other words, you can use your rig cage selectively. This brings you to a higher level of efficiency. For instance, as your self-awareness and relaxation skills improve, you will find that to achieve the total relaxation of the right arm, muscles around the right ribs should also be relaxed. Do not expect a big expansion of the ribs in the beginning, the ribs may move just a little bit. The important thing is the feeling of the expansion, the improvement in self-awareness, relaxation and isolation ability.

If you are an endurance sport athlete, the full thorax breathing technique is very important. The abdomen moving exercise may increase vital capacity by about 20%. The full thorax breathing technique may further increase the vital capacity by about another 10%. In this way, the intercostal muscle and the thoracic muscles are relaxed, a full breathing capacity is thus achieved. The congestion of the chest may no longer bother you. Since above the diaphragm, there are only the heart and the lungs. The increase in capacity will improve lung function and in turn improve normal heart function. The efficiency of your internal organs will improve. As a result, your endurance will improve.

Not only that, your voice will become full, rich and far-reaching. The breathing exercises deepen your respiration and strengthen your internal organs. The rib expanding exercises increase the flexibility and the relaxation of your upper body. All the exercises trains you to a total relaxed body. Therefore, in addition to a self-assured demeanor achieved, your voice will be full of confidence as well. This is why some people judge how well a person cultivates his internal body from his voice.

Furthermore, stronger muscles of the thoracic wall and a lower rate of ossification of rib cartilages obtained from these exercises will provide better prevention of internal injury.

Internal Center of Gravity Control

Experts define the diaphragm muscles as the primary respiratory muscles, like a singer needs. In Tai–ji fitness, the diaphragm muscles play additional important roles in both body control and explosive exertion. It is the most important part of the total body control and coordination. Therefore, I will introduce its beginning training and principles in detail here.

Our internal organs play a very important role in both health and sport. The internal organs takes a major portion of total body weight. Thus an ability to incorporate the internal movements into the external movements is essential.

In order for you to experience the subtleness and significance of internal center of gravity control, please try the following exercise:

Exercise 1: Spread your arms horizontally, stand on one leg, and lift the other to the side, then balance yourself as shown in Fig. 4–2. After you balance yourself with this posture, bring your internal organs up. You should notice that you fall automatically to the side. Have your hanging leg go across in front of you, and land to the side.

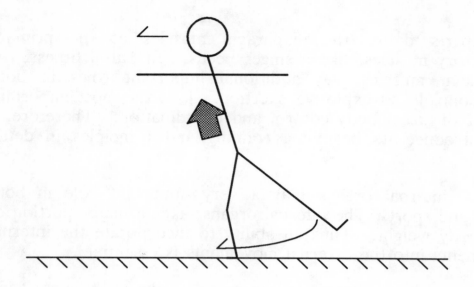

Figure 4–2 Internal Center of Gravity Control Exercise 1

Exercise 2: Lower your internal organs, then you will find yourself dropping back so that both feet are on ground as shown in Fig. 4–3.

Now you have experienced the effect of internal control. This is the key to precise body control. For example, gymnasts can use it to perfect their skills.

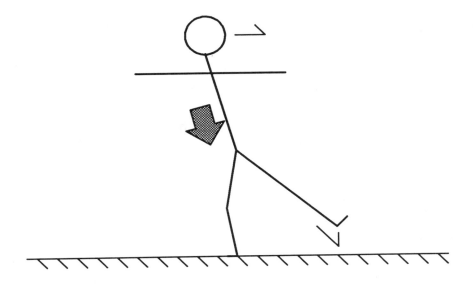

Figure 4-3   Internal Center of Gravity Control Exercise 2

A friend of mine who practices Tai-ji Quan told me of his experience. Once he went out to climb a mountain with his friends. On the way back down, he could not help rushing forward. This made it very hard for him to keep his balance. Then he recalled what he learned from Tai-ji Quan. He intentionally lowered his center of gravity by loosening up his lower abdomen. After doing so, it became much easier for him to keep his balance. Because he practices Tai-ji Quan, he was able to do so. This is very subtle. Yet, this is exactly the kind of things Tai-ji practitioners pursue.

111

Coordination of Internal and External Body

A story about another master is told as the follows: His father, a great martial artist once put him with his 10 senior students in a dark room. In less than a minute, he walked out from the room, leaving all others laying on the floor. He had always been very swift, light and fast. When he moved, his students noticed that his stomach moving in and out with his movements. What does this mean? This means that he has an excellent coordination of internal and external body.

After you have learned the abdomen moving skill, the following exercises train you how to use this skill in body movements and sports.

Knee rolling exercise: Adding the internal organ movements into the knee rolling exercise, when you draw a vertical circle with your two cooperated legs, as your body going down, lower your internal organs down accordingly, as your body going up, lift your internal organs up as well. I am telling you the direct phenomenon. If you have mastered the reversal breathing technique. It is easier not to think of your internal organs but simply inhale as you going up and exhale as you going down. Notice this when you practice the external knee exercise, if you keep your internal organs stiff, your body's external circular movement is also your center of gravity circular movement. After you master the knee rolling exercise, then you can try to practice this exercise with its real purpose, internal–external coordination. Moving your center of gravity in a smooth circle with the involvement of your internal organs.

Tango walk exercise: Do the Tango walk as described in previous section. Walk very slowly. When you begin to step forward, start to raise your center of gravity by lifting your internal organs higher. You should find that lifting the center of gravity higher makes the leg step out easily and lightly. The key here is to learn initiating movements from your internal organs. After the foot lands on the ground firmly, while shifting your weight forward to that leg, lower your center of gravity by dropping your internal organs to your lower abdomen. Your center of gravity in this whole process draws a line as shown in Fig. 4-4.

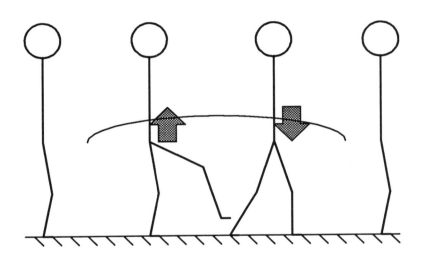

Figure 4-4 Internal Tango Walk Exercise

Half stepping exercise: Take a bow stance, make a half step, and lunge a push or a punch as shown in Fig. 4-5. When stepping the half step, lift your internal organs. In other words, initiate the movements from your internal organs. During the lunging, lower your internal organs, and at the same time, extend your hands out. Change the leg, and continue to do this until you feel comfortable with it. Note that if you practice fencing, you may alter this exercise a little bit by changing the arm and hand positions.

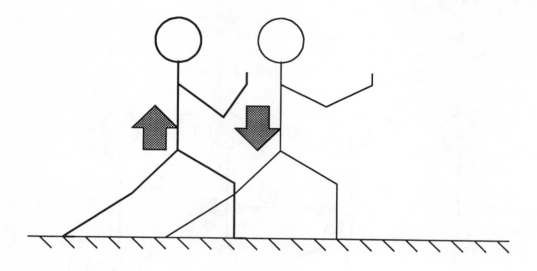

Figure 4-5 Half Stepping Exercise

Now let us use our imagination to analyze two persons who both have equal external muscles and other conditions, but one has a stiff stomach while the other has a strong and trained internal muscles which enables him to move with a subtle coordination between the external and the internal. Who has the better skill? I think the answer goes without saying. After the discussion above, I hope the skepticism toward the story told in the beginning of this section will be gone. I personally believe in it.

I hope that I have revealed some of the mystery of Tai-ji Quan. As long as one pursues one's sport with the Tao of Tai-ji, one will benefit from it. Many athletes today can get a gold medal without a good internal training. By looking at the developing history of Wu-shu, I predict that in the early 21st century it will become impossible to be a gold medalist without systematical internal training.

Running

Now that you have read all the basic skills introduced in this book, you can apply them to your favorite sports. In this section, I use running as an example to show you how to apply Tai-ji principles and techniques to aerobic exercises. If you do not run regularly, you may try one run first, remember the reactions of your body during and after the running. Stop running and do 3 weeks Tai-ji exercises. Then you may run again. Comparing your experiences from these two runs, you should feel a big difference. Here is how you do it.

Before running: Use the knee rolling exercise to improve your lower angle muscle strength and control. Runners usually do not need knee flexibility at small angles, they may have very flexible knees from 180 degrees (straight leg) to about 160 degrees. From 160 degrees and below, they have very poor control over their center of gravity. Practicing this exercise at lower angles will reduce the chance of suffering knee injuries, and improve your handling of down-hill running.

Do the shaking exercise to relax your body. Do the touching exercise to check each part of your body. Do the leg stretching exercise to stretch at all angles. Do the breathing exercises to stretch and relax your internal organs. Do the spine rocking exercise and the side reaching exercise to stretch and relax your spines. Do the shoulder rowing exercise to stretch and relax your upper body and shoulders. Do the rib expanding exercises to limber up your upper body and to relax your intercostal muscles, back muscles and chest muscles.

During running:
a) Keep your center of gravity at a relative constant level. Use the Tango walk skill.
b) Concentrate on your body. Constantly analyze yourself. Feel how each part of your body functions.
c) Be efficient. Use the skill learned from the leg swinging exercise.

d) Never go against your body. Be natural.

When running up—hill, use the skill learned from the ankle tilting exercise, distribute your weight evenly on your feet, do not use your balls only. In this way, your calf muscles will not be overstressed, so that you will not get pain on your calves after the running.

When running down—hill, use the skill learned from the Tango walk exercise, do not tense up your leg muscles suddenly, allow your knee to bend further to maintain the continuity of your body momentum.

After running: You should be energetic or feel a little bit tired. The tireness you get should be over after few minutes of meditation, or a nap. This indicates the changes in your body's metabolism are within the elasticity range of your body. If the tireness is not over in the next day or so, that means you overdid it. You should reduce the amount of exercises you do. If you feel pains, you should immediately stop the exercise.

Some people run until they feel short of breath and their heart is going to jump out of their throat. They think that is aerobic. This is wrong. Actually, they simply create chaos in their body. When the shortness of breath happens, this is an indication of disorder in their body's function and metabolism. Their body are abused and sabotaged, not strengthened and rejuvenated.

After practicing Tai—ji exercises, you will be able to tell how much is enough. However, this is not because I am smart to tell you all of this, and you will become smart after the practice of Tai—ji exercises. This is because our body is intelligent. Applying the self—awareness and flexibility developed from Tai—ji fitness exercises, you will enjoy your exercises and sports instead of suffer. Your fitness will improve in a steady pace. You will not complain that exercises give you fatigue not energy. This is the "Tao" of Tai—ji.

116

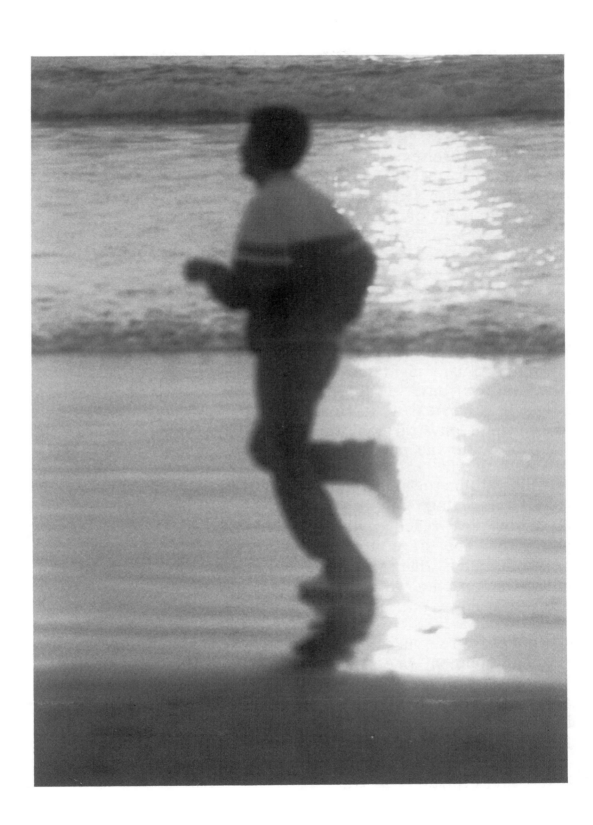

Some Personal Experiences

Tai—ji exercises are very effective in gaining inner energy or stamina, especially the exercises described in this basic internal training section. There are generally four stages in the development of Tai—ji fitness.

Stage 1: General physical condition improves. All problems and diseases are gone.
Stage 2: Attain some stamina and some flexibility. You are able to do your work every day without feeling tired in the evening.
Stage 3: Obtain some extra stamina. You can do exercises, go watch a late night movie, sleep less hours, without feeling tired the next day.
Stage 4: Gain extra stamina. Become very energetic. Be in an excellent physical condition. Feel like a child, you want to jump high, tumble on the ground, yell loudly and so on.

The key here is that do not get into competitive sports in stage 1 and stage 2. If you want to be competitive, to this after you have reached stage 3. The best way is to do it after you reach the stage 4. By that time, you will become so energetic such that you have to find a way to burn your energy. You then will be able to handle the intense training in a relaxed, enjoyable, injury—free and ease manner.

A person's success is directly related to his health. Without stamina, one has no courage to meet any challenge. Without stamina, one has very little chance to be successful in any field. Before my Tai—ji practice, I did exercise everyday in college, I got tired after 10 p.m., I had to go to bed. After I started Tai—ji practice, I rejuvenated my inner energy, I could stay late for home—work and studies, I could sleep better and efficiently as well.

At one time, I got locked out. My car was over 3 miles away from my house. It was winter in Minnesota. I had to go home to get the spare key. I started to run. At that time, I was busy with my Ph. D. thesis, my new job, and my baby. I had no time to do regular exercise for a long time. But I never stopped doing my Tai—ji exercises. I did them in my office, in my car, in any possible occasion available. When I hold my baby, I did the figure 8 shifting, the knee rolling and the hip circling exercises. So, my body quickly adapted to the running, soon my pace became steady. I got home without a stop. I ran back to my car with no feeling of out of breath and any discomfort. I was then further convinced the efficacy of my Tai—ji exercises.

You may do 100 sit—ups at a time and develop a firm stomach. Do you really feel healthier and stronger? In fact, you may still get tired easily. After you are on the way of Tai—ji fitness, you will find that you become healthier and stronger. You will enjoy your life more. You will feel confident, energetic and strong inside. You may find out what you did before is a bit superficial. Your strong appearance before was only skin—deep. You may be wondering how I know this. You may think I am laughing at you. You are wrong. I am laughing at myself many years ago. Of course, if your stomach muscles are weak, you need to do sit—up exercises first.

END

You may find that without pursuing what has been described here, you can still be a champion. This book is aimed to help you to further perfect your skills. History has proved that Tai-ji Quan is one of the best martial arts. The spirit of Tai-ji should be the spirit of Excellency today.

I do not consider myself as a martial artist. My martial art skill is poor. What I describe here is only the basic Tai-ji fitness requirements. It is perhaps only one sixth of the way to become a Tai-ji martial artist. But I do consider myself as a Tai-ji fitness artist. I hope now you have shared this experience with me.

Since Tai-ji exercises are detailed, this makes it more difficult to describe them in writing. Therefore, only the exercises, I consider being representative, are introduced. After you master them, you are ready to practice higher level, more comprehensive Tai-ji exercises. But the basic skills described in this book are mandatory to further pursue higher level Tai-ji fitness exercises. The principles have to be understood thoroughly. Therefore, I think this book will help you a great deal.

INDEX

About The Author

Dr. Zhang was born in Changchun, China, in 1957. He received the B.S. degree in Physics in 1982, from Peking University, Beijing, China, and his M.S. and Ph.D. degrees in Electrical Engineering from the University of Minnesota, Minneapolis, in 1983 and 1986, respectively.

In order to improve memory, concentration, productivity and stamina, Dr. Zhang started his pursuit of total fitness in 1978 after he suffered from chronic gastritis. Ever since then, the pursuit of total fitness became a project that went in parallel with his pursuit of career. He met Dr. David J. Wu in 1983 and studied Tai-ji Quan under Dr. Wu's special guidance for three years. He had also studied Tai-ji Quan with several other teachers. He visited many Tai-ji schools, martial arts studios and fitness clubs in the United States and learned and exchanged the knowledge of Tai-ji Quan and fitness with their instructors. Dr. Zhang is also a musician, and plays half dozen Chinese folk music instruments skillfully.

He is currently an electrical engineer, and has ten technical publications and several patents. His success today in engineering is inseparable from his pursuit of total fitness. He is currently living in San Diego, California, with his wife and two sons. He teaches Tai-ji Quan and especially Tai-ji Fitness Exercises in his spare time.